Mad Parts of Sane People in Analysis

Murray Stein, editor

Chiron Publications ● Wilmette, Illinois

The Chiron Clinical Series
ISBN 0-933029-67-5

General Editor: Murray Stein
Managing Editor: Siobhan Drummond
Book Review Editor: Laura McGrew

© 1993 by Chiron Publications. All rights reserved. No part of this publication may be reproduced, stored in a retrieval system, or transmitted in any form, by any means, electronic, mechanical, photocopying, recording, or otherwise, without the prior written permission of the publisher, Chiron Publications, 400 Linden Avenue, Wilmette, Illinois 60091.

Printed in the United States of America.

Book design by Elaine Hill.

Library of Congress Cataloging-in-Publication Data

Mad parts of sane people in analysis / Murray Stein, editor.
    p. cm. — (The Chiron clinical series)
    Includes bibliographical references.
    ISBN 0-933029-67-5 : $15.95
    1. Psychoanalysis. 2. Psychotherapy patients. 3. Psychology, Pathological. I. Stein, Murray, 1943– . II. Series.
RC506.M255 1993
616.89′14—dc20
                                     92-39057
                                         CIP
                                       Rev.

Contents

Jung, Madness and Sexuality: Reflections on Psychotic Transference and Countertransference

Introduction

The tendency in analysis to sidestep the act of experiencing and embracing psychotic aspects of a patient's personality is all too common. An analyst's desire to employ understanding and thus avoid the experience of emptiness and dissociative chaos is difficult to put aside. But Jung's psychology encourages us to do just that. Jung developed a system capable of filling up any void or absence with a mythologem or the knowledge that one exists even if unknown at the moment (Dehing 1990, Joseph 1987). But it is often precisely such experiences of absence of affect, and especially an absence of thinking, that reveal psychotic process. This is not to say that the unknowable, for example, the symbol or the archetype *per se*, doesn't play an important role in Jung's thought. But the overall spirit of his psychology is that knowledge exists which can put order into chaos.

In Jung's "Seven Sermons to the Dead," written near the end of his four-year descent into the unconscious and experience of psychotic

Nathan Schwartz-Salant, Ph.D., is a Jungian analyst, trained in Zürich, and in private practice in New York City. He is the author of *Narcissism and Character Transformation, The Borderline Personality: Vision and Healing*, and numerous clinical papers. He is president of the Salant Foundation and director of the Center for Analytical Perspectives.

© 1993 by Chiron Publications.

states after his break with Freud, emptiness is called the devil. Some thirty years later, while exploring the *Rosarium Philosophorum*, we find Jung regarding states of mind depicted in the seventh woodcut, known as the *Impregnatio* or the "Ascent of the Soul," as "defy[ing] our powers of scientific description" (1946b, par. 481) and that "the idea of mystery forces itself upon the mind of the inquirer (as) admission of his inability to translate what he knows into the everyday speech of intellect" (ibid.). But then knowledge quickly prevails, as evidenced by Jung's following remark: "I must content myself with the bare mention of the archetype which is inwardly experienced at this stage, namely the birth of the 'divine child' " (ibid.). This woodcut refers to states of splitting and absence, a deep level of *nigredo*, which is cloaked in mystery. It refers to a gap between humankind and the sacred that can be neither bridged nor understood and also refers to states of mind that preclude empathy. But in Jung's approach, the experience of the state of absence is barely valued; knowledge *about it* prevails.

Having discovered that he was not psychotic but rather in his own *nekyia*, and having seen the mysteries as did the mythical Jonah in the whale, Jung seemed to place a seal upon these depths which had provided him with the vision for all his future work.

> It all began then; the later details are only supplements and clarifications of the material that burst forth from the unconscious, and at first swamped me. It was the *prima materia* for a lifetime's work. (Jung 1961, p. 199)

Most Jungians have been trained to deal with his system as if Jung were the one to plunge into the depths, mine the ore, and offer us the work of cleaning and polishing it. Jung warned all away from these depths, save those individuals with, as he put it, a certain moral strength of character. He regarded his explorations as not only his *prima materia* but that of his students as well. This was not one of his more fortunate attitudes.

Mad Parts of Sane People

A sane person's mad or psychotic parts are those aspects of psyche that are not contained by the self and for which the psyche's self-regulating function fails. The self represents those aspects of the Self, the larger totality of personality, that have been integrated, being both a center and a containing circumference for the ego. This experience of containment expands with personality integration. But the psychotic parts of a personality always are at the edge of this self structure, at best a boundary phenomenon and at worst ever-intruding, disrupting any felt sense of containment. These psychotic parts, like the chaotic waters of mythology, are part of the Self; they are always crucial to change and regeneration.

Speaking about a psychotic part is, in a sense, a contradiction. One never experiences psychotic states in another person as if they were a part of the person, as we sometimes speak of a complex. Psychotic states, like the waters of chaos in alchemy or in creation myths, are psychic spaces in which Cartesian language fails. These states readily extend to the analyst, creating a field in which it is not possible to state who is containing "the psychotic part." Rather, one deals with a field phenomenon that cannot be reduced to separable structures. Generally, the term *psychotic part* or a similar word is meant here as shorthand to help designate that domain of experience in which psychotic process dominates. It does not indicate an approach in which one speaks of "a patient's psychotic part" as if it were in any manner totally separable from the same phenomenon in the analyst. Rather, transference psychosis constellates countertransference psychosis, but in a lesser degree and a more manageable form, that is, if the analysis of these areas is to be successful.

I would like to note the peculiar nature of the opposites as they are often encountered in the psychotic part. As later clinical material will exemplify, the opposites are not only split but each has a peculiar kind of wholeness to it. I am not referring here to the so-called primary process that dominates part-objects; rather, each opposite can act as a mirror and the split encountered may be thought of as a split mirror, with each reflection demanding to be totally embraced.[1] Consequently, if one senses a dark, psychopathic quality and mirrors it, either empathically or interpretively, one will meet a strong resistance. In turn, one may discover and mirror a split opposite, e.g., a very creative or even numinous part, and encounter the same resistance. It is as if seeing one part is always experienced as not seeing by the patient, whether the part seen is positive or negative, and it is extremely difficult to get these opposites together. My experience with this leads me to believe that the opposites involved are those of life and death, and the patient knows, in a deep preconscious way, that he or she has to get them together. Thus, seeing something extremely positive in the person is not helpful without seeing the opposite, yet each opposite can demand being seen as total. This makes for a difficult clinical experience, but it is one that can only be embraced if it is just that, *an experience* for both patient and analyst.

In analytical work, when the psychotic sector is enlivened, a transference emerges akin to the psychotic transference with schizophrenic patients as described by Searles. The transference "distorts or prevents a relatedness between patient and therapist as two separate, alive, human and sane beings" (Searles 1965, p. 669). The difference between the psychotic transference with the schizophrenic person and the constellation of this sector in a nonpsychotic person is one of degree and structure. It engulfs the schizophrenic, but it is partially held out by splitting defenses when it is a mad part of a normal person.

When defenses such as denial, idealization, and mind–body splitting begin to fail, the psychotic parts intrude into the conscious personality. The person becomes highly dissociated and can oscillate between phases of unreality in relationship to his or her own person and to others. Behavior and fantasy stemming from these parts can distort reality in very subtle ways. The person may behave in ways that he or she thinks are inspired but, in fact, are psychopathic, with absolutely no regard for another person or his or her own soul. The analyst is commonly affected in similar ways. When a patient's madness emerges in an analysis, the therapist will often feel disoriented and find it extremely difficult to concentrate and contain the process at hand. One's own center seems to fail and bizarre objects dominate (Grotstein 1990).

When the psychotic part projects onto an object or dominates the organization of the subject's inner world, it distorts reality. Such states are created by the simultaneity of totally conflicting messages. While the "double bind," in which different messages are given in succession or in which mind and body offer conflicting messages, is a good example of such a conflict, the experience one has when the psychotic part of a normal person is constellated is usually more subtle. Images of a usually malevolent nature arise and combine with qualities of a personal parental figure, often yielding bizarre objects that seem to defy understanding. When a person begins to integrate his or her psychotic part, that person's normal ego-consciousness is expanded but in an unsettling way, for the ego knows that here it is not in control of its thoughts and behavior. The feeling tone of the psychotic part attempts to signal the ego that it could act in very destructive ways *within the delusion of being in control*. In a sense, the psychotic part is an open wound that breeds delusion, but when the ego accepts both the limitation of its consciousness *and* of its own capacity for control, it can produce a caring attitude for soul. As Lacan (1977) said, "Not only can man's being not be understood without madness, it would not be man's being if it did not bear madness within itself as the limit of his freedom."

Dionysus and the Psychotic Part

I include the following reflections on the Greek god Dionysus for several reasons. The phenomenology of this god has remarkable similarities with the psychotic part of a normal person. We can learn a great deal from the Greek experience, or at least attune ourselves to listening in ways that are not bound by developmental constructs. While it is often possible to understand the psychotic part in its formation and dynamics from early developmental failures (and this understanding is essential), it can become too small a container. Like the "neither-nor logic" (Schwartz-Salant 1989) that applies to this part, and to which we shall later return in more detail, this phenomenon is neither created, for example, by early trauma, nor is it not created. It is neither a *creatum* nor an *increatum*. It is neither archetypal nor is it developmental in nature. We are dealing with a paradox in which both possibilities exist, defying a clear-cut differentiation. Dealing with the psychotic part demands the capacity to tolerate the ambiguity of its peculiar logic, which causes a suspension of the either-or certainty of discursive reasoning processes. But this does not exclude the possibility such reasoning may, so to speak, fall out of the experience of this part.

For what follows, I will call upon works on Dionysus by Detienne (1989), Otto (1965), Hillman (1972), Kerenyi (1976), and Paglia (1990). Dionysus is an excellent mythological example of the nature of the mad part of a normal personality. This part can be denied if we live only from a mental–spiritual vantage point as represented by an Olympian god such as Apollo. Then we may reckon its manifestation as creating hysteria, which would be to misunderstand Dionysus. The psychotic part, like Dionysus, creates a sense of strangeness: we don't know the person when this part is constellated, and he or she only marginally knows us. We call this the psychotic transference, but that is an Apollonian approach to naming an experience that feels weird, strange.

Dionysus corresponds to a feeling level that has both mystery and danger in it. The psychotic part, with its split opposites, gives forth a sense of emptiness, of being deadened. Yet when these opposites are brought together, the experience shifts to one of fullness. Dionysus combines such states of absence and presence. The person we see, when the psychotic part is enlivened, always wears a mask. We see a stranger, someone we truly do not know, and the strangeness is unsettling. But like the experience of Dionysus, there are two masks, two strangers, one seeming to pull toward life and fullness, the other toward death and deadness.

We cannot see this unless we look through our own psychotic part, i.e., through the felt experience of limitation by our own madness. This is a sacrifice to the god, as the Greeks put it, an *epidemic* in which we participate when he appears through our patient. For those who know their own defilement through madness, he becomes a purifying god. This is an essential issue when it comes to relating to mad parts, for the analyst must know ways in which he or she has defiled another soul through acts that were either blatantly destructive at the time or, more to the point, acts that were driven secretly by a hidden madness. Such behaviors often take the form of intrusion or withdrawal, based upon a belief in one's sane, courageous behavior which dares to break with conventional wisdom. Yet later one learns that the actions in question were mad and highly destructive. All instances of sexual acting out in psychotherapy fall under this category of madness. At the time, the analyst really believes he or she is sane and serving special energies. People who have succumbed in this way will often speak of feeling that a higher power was being served and to do otherwise would have been a form of cowardice and failure.

But Dionysus, in fact, does not demand that one become mad, only that one acknowledge madness! It is a form of respect; one follows him when he appears. He becomes purifying to those who know they are up against a border of knowledge and being in which they do not have the capacity to know if they are mad or not. Respecting the power of such unknowing respects the god, while acting in mad ways does not. In Greek myth those who became mad after rejecting his rites, committing horrendous acts such as child murder, are themselves shunned and dismembered. Thus, it is the awareness of our serious failures, defilements of soul, and a capacity to carry this history and speak and be with it as alive, within us, that creates the voice tone and feeling through which a patient's psychotic part can be known and accepted. We may, through rational understanding that appeals to the patient's normal-neurotic side, deny Dionysus, and as a consequence madness will take its toll as severe dissociation and a brutal attack upon one's inner life. Such states of mind are usually felt by the patient as the analyst subtly withdraws and gives the message that one does not want his or her madness in the room. Dionysus is not one to forgive slights, even when attempts are quickly made to change one's attitude. Manic defenses emerge, and the patient will tend toward drugs or food to sooth the inner rage that is unbearable and destructive.

Dionysus is a god who leads large-scale invasions that spread among people: he is contagious just as the psychotic part is known to be in psychic infection. He causes us to stumble and to create a new view of life. We are called upon to build our images of a psyche anew, and to do so immediately. This is how the psychotic part affects one, if its opposites are held together and if its ferocity is respected.

When we encounter the opposites in their split form, we meet Dionysus in his most deathlike aspect, as Paglia says, "in the long slow suck, the murk and ooze" (1990, p. 6). We feel this in the interactive field. There is no heart, no spontaneity, but rather a sense of alienation, deadness, emptiness, and, if we look further, the ever-present sense of strangeness. We may speak of a derealized-depersonalized sequence: Apollonian talk. Good talk. But what we know is an uncomfortable feeling: the person is strange to us and we are strange to ourselves.

There is a murderer in Dionysus, and a murderer in the psychotic part. There resides a person's psychopathy in the form of a total lack of concern for us, a ruthlessness that knows no compassion. Yet, do we ever meet this part by interpreting it to the patient? No matter what we do along the way, no matter how we inwardly experience the contagion of the god, and no matter how we frame this in an interpretation, we have still shifted levels, gone from Dionysus to Apollo. All this does is yield a knowledge that represses, not a living knowledge of the way we are forever limited by our madness. How then is the patient to know this part? Only by being *known* through it in ourselves, only by being known in his or her strangeness, known in the felt moment of an interactive field. And moreover, the patient will see our psychopathy, will know such parts in us, and when this can be acknowledged, then he or she can dare accept these parts within himself or herself.

We do not deal here with a mere conscious–unconscious split, but one that also includes a radical separation of opposites within the complex itself. It is this split that we encounter within the interactive field, while conscious–unconscious repression can be employed to deny its pain and sense of strangeness. This split can also be employed to deny the powers involved. Dionysus is a bull, a panther. Such wild energies inhabit the psychotic part and can be known when seen as such, when the defenses of idealization and dissociation are successfully gathered up and dissolve. Yet when the opposites are finally held together, distance gives way to closeness, emptiness to fullness, and a containing heart develops where the felt experience of the heart with oneself or the other had previously been absent.

The word *psychosis* comes from the Greek, where it means "soul animation." At root, this is what we are after, the animation of a soul that has been frozen in early terrifying experiences of chthonian life. A succinct and vivid account of this level is offered by Camille Paglia in her book *Sexual Personae*:

> What the West represses in its view of nature is the chthonian, which means "of the earth" — but earth's bowels, not its surface. . . . I adopt it as a substitute for Dionysian, which has become contaminated with vulgar pleasantries. The Dionysian is no picnic. It is the chthonian realities which Apollo evades, the blind grinding of subterranean force, the long slow, suck, the murk and ooze. It is the dehumanizing brutality of biology and geology, the Darwinian waste and bloodshed, the squalor and rot we must block from consciousness to retain our Apollonian integrity as persons. . . . The daemonism of chthonian nature is the West's dirty little secret. (Paglia 1990, p. 5f)

Paglia's passionate book is a powerful corrective to all those who idealize the Dionysian and the chthonian level, or who believe it can be transformed. Rather, it transforms us, works upon us as we are its object. It is the chaos that can become order but always remains dangerous and bloody.

In their fullness, the Dionysian energies have always been felt as dangerous in their flooding capacity. To partake of these energies constructively, one must learn of the power and danger of the chthonic realm and of its fundamental otherness to the ego. In the Attis mysteries, the initiates, during the ritual of the Taurobolean, lay beneath a grid atop which a bull was sacrificed. Fifty liters of blood rushed over those below (Burkert 1987, p. 98). If ever there was a ritual which provided one with the experience of the difference between one's mortal being and the powers of the chthonic archetype, this kind of archaic sacrifice surely provides it.

Nowadays, the chthonic life of the body is mostly taken for granted. A person's sexuality is generally considered to be contained within the individual as a biological drive, while the *numinosum* is usually reserved for a spiritual, disembodied world. But sexuality is a daemon, an archetypal power whose numinosity is only thinly veiled in modern culture. Freud's insistence upon the sexual basis of internal fantasy life, although representing a one-sided point of view, accounts in large measure for why he continues to be taken seriously.

Gathering Up the Psychotic Transference

Analysts all have different ways of dealing with the dynamics of the psychotic transference. But when the analyst's attention begins to fragment, and states of inner deadness, emptiness, and confusion emerge, what can contain such states? An act of will, for example, an intense concentrated effort, can often embrace a schizoid withdrawal or the regression accompanying the disturbed equilibrium of the narcissistic character. But the dissociation from the psychotic part generally overpowers the analyst's ego. Often, but not always, a containing quality can come from the analyst's awareness that a psychotic transference is working behind the scenes. The patient may be quite rational and connected to affects, unlike the splitting dynamics in a schizoid state, but the person is dominated by a projection of a psychotic nature. From the point of view of this sector, the analyst is a dangerous, persecutory object; the as-if of a nonpsychotic projection is lost. Furthermore, it is the *way we see* this state that is of the essence if the psychotic part is to be contained. It must be known by the analyst as a psychic reality, but also as an imaginal presence that the analyst experiences in a just-so, embodied way. When we see the psychotic part, the tendency is to recoil from its reality-distorting nature which sees us as someone completely different from who we are. The patient feels strange to us. This is inherent in the phenomenology of madness as it erupts into one's normal everyday world; as we have noted, it is part of the god Dionysus, but it is also an enactment of the patient's fear of being seen as a psychic leper. One must, consequently, be able to see the psychotic part in a matter-of-fact way: here is a wounded and limited person (as we all are), but still someone of beauty and value, much of which is, in fact, a result of suffering the psychotic level.

Often, if the analyst loses an embodied, down-to-earth state and then *talks about* the reality distortions of the psychotic transference, the patient can recognize that what is said is correct, but dissociative states will return to both of them because containment of the anxiety fails. However, if interpretation is made while the analyst remains embodied, while actively experiencing and envisioning the psychotic sector, interpretation can be very containing to the patient. The psychotic transference is a state in which some degree of analyst–patient alliance still exists. Hence, when the analyst is able to *see* the patient's distrustful double, something in the patient is relieved and a sense of containment ensues. In contrast, when the quality of patient–analyst alliance vanishes and the transference becomes delusional, no amount of vision or empathic connection or understanding has a containing influence. Instead, one remains, at least for the time being, in a state where the devil has gained the upper hand.

Manifestations of the Psychotic Part

The following list is a series of signposts to aid the therapist in containing the psychotic field. The mad part, at its core, breaks up thoughts, leads to states of blankness, and especially afflicts the patient with mental torment in which anything he or she feels or thinks can readily be undone, leading to a state in which what was said has no meaning at all. The patient realizes that he or she has been grasping for straws in a vacuum, with absolutely no sense at all of an inner orientating center or background support to give a sense of being on the right track. Instead, no track is meaningful.

Here one approaches experiences not only of being overwhelmed, but of states that can be called neither mental nor physical. Rather, they are both and are most poignantly known in a sense of pain that feels boundless. Many experience this pain in the chest area, as a state in which the Other—person or god—is absent. Instead, there is nothing but an agony of dread, an experience bordering on nonexperience which leads many to believe that they are, in this awful inner hell, afflicted by unassimilated feelings and perceptions of a lifetime. These nonmetabolized states occur with no images, just pain and terror for their seeming endlessness. This level recalls Jung's notion of the psyche as extending along states bounded by the "psychoid level," on the one end the infrared of instinctual and somatic process, and on the other end the ultraviolet of mental and spiritual process (Jung 1946a, par. 420). At the psychotic level, these opposites fuse in an undifferentiated way or were never separate.

When the psychotic level is sufficiently gathered up, it becomes evident just how an absence of bonding opens the gates to the terror of this level. I think it is wrong to say it "causes" this level to exist, because such domains are archetypal, prior to creation in the sense of temporally acquired structures or the absence of what should have developed. But bonding problems are especially evident in the degree of lack of containment that the psychotic level ushers into the ego's awareness.

An especially important quality that comes into play as a result of bonding problems is a very deep masochism. The person reacts to the black hole of psychosis (Grotstein 1990) with a black sponge of masochism. To counteract the void of bonding, the person bonds with everything that he or she feels as wrong, whatever wrong might be. Everything from the slightest shifts of interest or attention on the part of the object, real or distorted through paranoid process, to outright attacks of guilt by the object are absorbed on a very deep level. This is a core phenomenon of the psychotic part, and one of the horrors of this dynamic is that it proceeds quite autonomously. To treat this level of masochism as the "scapegoat" is far too sophisticated; this kind of word magic blunts the horror of the fact that, at some point, we are all sponges for anything we perceive as dark or wrong. The person with a strong psychotic part is utterly ruled by this state. He or she bonds through it, a masochistic bond in which contact with another person is not felt, but instead the pain of noncontact takes its place. To actually bond in a genuine way would require trusting another person at this level, a situation that is totally alien and only becomes an image and a possibility once the psychotic level has been exposed and contained.

The psychotic part manifests in myriad ways, but the following list of relatively common phenomena provides a map of a territory. (Clearly, as is often emphasized, the map is not the territory.) Perceiving these features requires that the analyst register and use countertransference.

1. Dissociation

The analyst experiences a tendency to dissociate. This can include the withdrawal and energy loss common to schizoid dynamics, but primarily it is a state of fragmentation in which it is extremely difficult to concentrate on the patient. Feelings of emptiness, absence, mindlessness, and deadness can emerge. Any attempt at a fixed orientation easily falters and tends to shift to an opposite. As a consequence of these uncomfortable states of mind, hatred of the patient and a tendency to withdraw or attack can be felt.[2]

The analyst tends to avoid making affective contact with the patient at these times, especially by splitting from negative feelings. Instead, the dissociation is allowed to pass, going on as if nothing had happened. A concomitant tendency, which is often diagnostic of the constellation of the psychotic part, is that the analyst begins to stress the patient's strengths and address the normal-neurotic part. It may be later learned that the analyst, through this maneuver, has been stressing one of the opposites in the psychotic part and excluding another in hopes of reducing the anxiety he or she feels.

2. The Transference

If the analyst successfully encounters the dissociative field, maintains a cohesive presence, and "feels into" the patient, the field begins to clarify from a welter of attacking, image-destroying fragments to actual images. It is at this point that the analyst may recognize the psychotic transference. Not uncommonly, the analyst is viewed, through the patient's psychotic sector, as an attacking animal or as a dangerous parental figure. Often, the analyst becomes identified with those parts of the parental psyche that were especially dangerous to the patient. An example is seeing the analyst as dead, a state that can later be discovered to have been part of a parent's psychotic inner life which the patient splits off from awareness. As part of the clarification of the psychotic transference, the analyst senses that he or she is being seen in an extremely unreal way. The patient at these times also seems odd or strange to the analyst, for the psychotic state so opposes the normal-neurotic part one would rather experience. If one succeeds in comprehending this transference, it often becomes clear that, along with a sense that the analyst is not quite the analyst previously known, the patient also feels very strange to himself or herself.

3. Resistance

Along with this derealized-depersonalized sequence, the patient's resistances to experiencing the psychotic part become much clearer. These resistances commonly are of an erotic, compulsive, manic, or sadomasochistic nature. For example, extreme forms of sadomasochism may have been split off into the psychotic part. When this part is contained and becomes embodied, it can become clear that much sado-masochistic behavior, such as extreme giving of oneself to others while also subtly withdrawing, is actually a defense against madness. It is also my impression that the experience of sexual abuse in one's early life resides in a psychotic sector, and recovering such memories requires working with the dynamics of this part.

4. Opposites

It often takes considerable time and effort to achieve consciousness of the distinct opposites within the psychotic sector. Generally, such opposites have the peculiar quality of being both totally split and fused: they seem to fly apart, but their distinctness vanishes. This recalls the nature of the alchemical Mercurius, who provides a good image of the field qualities that these opposites engender. Within this field, the analyst tends to feel identified with one or the other opposite but also tends to split off from experiencing the opposites. This peculiar combination of fusion and splitting places the opposites at the boundary that the alchemists referred to as occurring prior to the second day, i.e., before the separation of opposites. They emerge, separate, and then quickly fuse back into a merged, nondistinct state. Most important, in the psychotic part, fusion and separation of opposites can occur with extreme rapidity, and the ensuing oscillation creates panic and confusion.

Idealization plays an especially important role in the dynamics of the psychotic part. It is employed with extreme tenacity to block experiencing hatred and rage toward an object and to maintain an ideal self image. One patient, working with her psychotic part, when her idealizing defenses began to diminish, dreamed of a blinding light that quickly shifted into total blackness. These opposites rapidly oscillated, creating fear and panic and causing her to attempt to restore her idealizing defenses. Another patient began to hallucinate having the teeth of an animal, and on several occasions I have seen dream imagery or actual waking hallucinations in which the patient has animal claws. When these terrifying states are lived with and contained—i.e., not acted out with another person in, for example, extreme anger—then the opposites in the psychotic part can transform. Inanimate objects become animate, cold-blooded animal forms progress to warm-blooded ones, and animals transform to have partialèy human form or speech, to mention several examples.

The process of discovering the opposites in the psychotic part generally follows from experiencing them as extremely split within an interactive field and at times felt in projective identification. Each vies for the total attention of the analyst, and the gap engenders a state of absence or void in which one's energies are dulled and consciousness is difficult to maintain. When the opposites are apprehended as a related pair, which occurs when the analyst becomes capable of not identifying with either of the pair, a new development is possible. A union field can emerge, a felt experience of *coniunctio*. Through this experience, the heart center for both analyst and patient becomes more open. This is usually a new experience for the patient, for whom the experience and vision of the heart has usually been closed off by strong armoring. Even when this experience is not attained, apprehending the opposites can lead to a new consciousness of the psychotic sector, especially its limiting nature. One learns about its power to distort reality ever so subtly, and a process develops in which aspects of the psyche hidden within the psychotic sector emerge. Most commonly found is a schizoid part, whose essential weakness—lack of connection—and distorting nature leads to a profound sense of humiliation. Only the awareness of opposites as part of the ensuing consciousness allows this experience to be contained rather than turning into a persecutory state. As a result, what appears as schizoid and lifeless often begins to show itself as part of a highly energized field that has been split off. In such typical ways, the discovery of the psychotic part and working with its energies is akin to a process of creation.

5. Defenses

The opposites within the psychotic sector appear in a dynamic form related to the particular defensive structure that accompanies the psychotic part. For example, when the defense is narcissistic, the opposites will often appear as a split mirror. Each opposite behaves like the grandiose, exhibitionistic self. If the analyst is careful, however, it is possible to discern that each opposite isn't as whole as this dynamic can lead one to believe. One tends to see the patient, for example, as creative rather than psychopathic (or, alternatively, as psychopathic rather than creative) in order to avoid feeling mad and seeing the patient's madness. But once this pitfall is avoided, it becomes clear that one is actually engaging a split, and that each opposite does not have a primary-process quality of wholeness.

When the narcissistic level of defense has sufficiently dissolved, or if it was never a major factor, the opposites take on a different dynamic. While each still masquerades as whole, the split mirror quality—a felt demand to adhere totally to one or the other—diminishes. Instead, there is a tendency to withdraw and not see the opposites, which would bring into focus the weakness of the schizoid ego and, with it, a humiliated state that the patient has attempted to hide. Furthermore, it brings into focus a high level of paranoia.

In the case of the borderline structure, which can appear mad enough in its own right and is a largely defensive structure, the rapidly oscillating opposites in the psychotic part are masked. The rather stable "good–bad" splitting of the borderline masks the nature of the opposites in the psychotic part. But when this splitting collapses, the psychotic part is quite evident. When the borderline structure is more fragmented with a multiplicity of psychic centers, it still masks the psychotic part, for each center has a quality of wholeness to it, different from the feigned wholeness exhibited by each opposite in the psychotic part. In the borderline organization, a primary-process quality rules, and each psychic center functions as a whole. The ego alternately identifies with various centers as a form of flight from abandonment; as if chased by persecutory anxiety, it takes up housing in various places. Once the analyst thinks he or she understands the person's plight, the "house" becomes unsafe and the chase is on, leading to humorous anecdotes about the borderline, such as Searle's statement that he feels outnumbered. But the psychotic part is not ruled by the same kind of primary process. Each opposite does not really feel whole. Instead, this "wholeness" is compulsively sought out in order to bring understanding to the pain the psychotic part engenders.

6. "Neither-Nor" Logic

There is a peculiar "neither-nor" logic to the psychotic part. This is the logic that can also be discerned in the depths of the borderline organization and is accounted for there by the existence of the psychotic part. For example, a woman who had successfully worked through a number of defenses hiding the psychotic part, notably idealization, spoke of not feeling dead, but also not feeling alive. She said she did not feel full, nor did she feel empty. It was clearly not possible to say that anything she was feeling was definitive; rather, any quality was felt within a bewildering state of being neither X nor not X.

One runs into this most forcefully in the attempted recollections of incest among abuse victims. The person will usually be tormented by the question: "Did it or didn't it happen?" Or "Am I making this all up?" But whatever occurred emerges first out of a psychotic sector, and there one can only experience that it neither happened nor did it not happen. Suspension rules, a state severely opposed by paranoid mechanisms, which cannot tolerate ambiguity. Yet the analyst must be able to contain the question of whether it happened or not by tolerating just such a state of ambiguous suspension.

It is especially important that, having apprehended the opposites, a person can learn to respect the existence of the psychotic part and change accordingly. Psychologically, a sacrifice is involved, an awareness of being limited by its existence. In analysis, the therapist must submit to the state of being limited, especially by the "neither-nor" logic and extreme splitting in the psychotic part, states of mind which thoroughly challenge any of the analyst's feelings of omnipotence. But through this acceptance of limitation, a sense of an inner structure of self and an inner life of soul emerges, for both analyst and patient. Furthermore, one learns that the energies of the psychotic part have a strange capacity to open the heart, that to live near them is to create a heart-centered consciousness in which the imaginal realm is a powerful psychic reality and a means of "seeing" that was previously foreclosed.

The psychotic part and the transference it creates can thus be gathered up. To achieve this, working through the dynamics I have enumerated, must be practiced over and over again, for the Mercurial nature of the psychotic part induces attention and consciousness to slip away from its turmoil and depth. But continual effort leads to a relative stability in accessing this part of the patient, a situation that depends not only upon the archetypal dynamics of the psychotic level but also upon the analyst's willingness to access his or her own psychotic states of mind continually. When the transference and countertransference are gathered up, the patient will experience a degree of containment that enables a deeper nature of the psychotic part to be faced.

If the therapist can contain the psychotic part by recognizing both its existence and the total despair that patient suffers by believing it will never change, knowing also that the patient may be right but respecting the possibility that something may fall into or emerge out of this state, then a new self experience can come into existence. In a sense, the analyst sacrifices omnipotence and aligns with the patient's reality, because it may well be true. This is not a matter of mere empathy, but one of the courage to leave open the possibility of failure. All the analyst can really offer is a measured uncertainty in the face of the patient's pessimism. The mystery is that this is often enough, if the analyst also recognizes the patient's madness. Unless this is communicated, the analyst's not knowing will fail to have a creative edge.

An Example of the Psychotic Part and the Psychotic Transference

A person's madness is often deeply hidden and exposes itself only near the fringes of our image of the person. The following example illustrates this, as well as some defenses against the integration of the psychotic part, their resolution, and the process of this sector becoming an inner, psychic reality.

A patient sent me an article she had written; she had sent to others as well and was especially proud of having produced it. The next session, she asked: "What did you think of what I wrote?" She wondered if I had thought of phoning her or perhaps sending her a note after I had read it to give her some feedback. When she asked her question, I felt somewhat uncomfortable and found myself answering quite readily, replying that I found it moving and special. But I then wondered if she was talking about manners or empathy, or if she was demanding some response out of a sense of entitlement? All of these possibilities seemed to exist simultaneously. My answer did not satisfy her. It was not that, in itself, it failed; rather, she was upset that I had not called her or written to her immediately after I had read it. At this point, my own reality sense began to waver: Why hadn't I called? Was I being withholding? I began to ask her questions and, in great distress, she cried out that my questioning was driving her crazy. I replied that I probably wanted to drive her crazy because I was feeling driven crazy by her.

In the next session, the patient returned to her complaint of my lack of empathy. She said I had been inwardly dead and that I had consequently not been able or willing to give her what she needed. A sense of unreality crept over me; when she said "give her what she needed," I could not quite believe what I was hearing, it felt so odd to me. I had known elements of this state with her previously, but it was never so pronounced, and I sidestepped them by attempting to connect with her. But now I wondered if she really believed I was there to gratify her fantasies totally? Yes, she did believe this. My sidestepping response had reinforced this belief and further energized the power of her psychotic part. She felt that anything less demonstrated my failure in empathy. Who was I for her?[3]

Might I have handled this interaction differently? For example, should I have more forcefully and earlier interpreted the transference in which I was treated as her servant? But this kind of fusion state was absolutely necessary for the patient. From her perspective, she felt a desperate need for me to agree with her perceptions. And if I might have reflected this to her by crafting an interpretation (amply noting present-day and genetic factors) that, in essence, would have said: "You need me to see it in your way," this would have been experienced as intolerably distancing. It would only have reversed the master–slave polarity in the psychotic part and left her feeling totally vulnerable. If I had interpreted this way, there could have been two outcomes. It could have resulted in a split from the psychotic part and a flight toward ego functioning and a reenergizing of her narcissistic-defensive structure. Or, it could have energized the split master–slave polarity in a way in which I would have become the sadistic master, overwhelming her perception and highly energizing the psychotic transference. This would have been very treatment-destructive, for it would have replicated relationships that had brought her into treatment with me.

I chose neither of these paths, although it was difficult to restrain myself. Her mad control of me aroused my anger, and it was tempting to stay my confusion by such interpretations. But I was also helped by occasional positive feelings for her, like flowers that emerge from hardened earth. Also, I had a sense of her suffering of which I was aware even in our first session, and this awareness remained more or less continuous.

After this session, I felt conflicted. If I followed her script, I would have fused with her and mirrored her need, helping to create the experience of a deeply attuned, empathic mother that she so sorely lacked, a mother that saw the bigness and beauty of her soul even amidst her omnipotent demands. Her childhood experience was of a mother who provided little containment. Instead, she knew but tried to split from and deny the reality of feeling frightened of her mother, for at times she sensed her mother's rage and its sense of randomness. A child must deny the truth of such sight, for such vision leads to anxiety that is too overwhelming. As she explained how she wanted me to act, I felt unreal and experienced her as unreal as well, a depersonalized-derealized sequence that empathy perhaps could erase. So why hold back? Was not following her script, I wondered, a countertransference reaction, a meanness of spirit that wanted to rub her nose in reality? Was my sense that I would lie and be unreal if I did as she wanted only my own defense against having the kind of fantasy that she has? Was my own early trauma of disappointment so great that I do not dare to have such wishes and demands and hate her for having them, perhaps spoil them for her? There must have been some of this present, for I did not feel easy with her; I felt some tightness and anger at what I felt as her driving me crazy.

During the next session, she began with a complaint, which was unusual for her, stating that in previous times, when she spoke about another person, I had not recognized that she was really speaking about our process. This led me to think about these occurrences, and I imaginally re-created the feelings I had when she previously brought such complaints. It became clear that, at these times, if I had reflected her anxiety as concerning our work together, I would have opposed an implicit injunction from her which insisted that our work was fine. But if I had sided with that reaction, I would have been rejecting her perceptions—as contained in her messages about other people—that our work was problematic. The result of feeling these unconnected, conflicting states of mind was that I began to feel dull, inwardly deadened. As I told her about the opposite states I was experiencing, my head swayed from side to side, and she said, "So that's what's happening when you move your head like that!" She had noticed this for some time during our work but never called it to my attention because all her efforts were at holding herself together. By moving my head from side to side, she felt I was scrutinizing her. She found my facial expression labored, serious, and pained. Apparently, I had long felt this conflict but had not brought it to consciousness until this time. She could appreciate that she had created situations which were well-nigh impossible to react to simply.

It became clear why meeting her need for heightened enthusiasm over what she had written was so difficult. Within her there was another state of mind, expecting exactly the opposite, total rejection. That state would have been denied by empathizing with her mirroring needs. That is, not seeing this side of her would have been just as denying of who she was as would have been granting her wish for bountiful praise.

One might think that my inability to understand empathically her pain at not being seen and understood was the necessary material with which to work, rather than focusing upon her mad parts which operated through omnipotence and reality-denying idealizations. Why not, one might ask, respond as follows: "I am finding it difficult to feel connected to what you need. I wonder if you are also sensing and suffering a lack of feeling, an inner resource to see and contain you." In other words, why not address my felt lack of empathy? However, if I had proceeded in this way, I would have filled the void of nonlinking by providing a substitute for my lack of empathy through acknowledging that lack. I would have then reestablished myself as a selfobject, and the madness in which she was actually enveloped would not have been dealt with. Such mirroring would only have preserved the prior equilibrium she had maintained through splitting from the psychotic nature of her fusion demands.

During the ensuing sessions I continuously had to rediscover my point of view, as her insistence that I was poorly attuned to her not only had some merit but was communicated through a dissociative field created by her unintegrated psychotic parts. But the holding power of such doubts would pass as I was able to become more embodied and present to myself, and I would again intervene with the thought that an element of madness had taken over the session in which she had complained of my response to her article. I would then further interpret that denying this was a way of re-creating her old form of equilibrium through finding a way to idealize me.

As a result of this working-through process, she came to the point of realizing not only the difference between feeling a need and having it met, but that her madness was a part of her. Previously, she only knew this as an overwhelming anxiety that was outside of her and afflicted her at times. Her defense was to become rigidly compulsive, aggressive, and withdrawn. This madness would then pass, like a storm, until the next time. But knowing it as an inner reality led to a fundamental change in her perception of herself. In fact, a self emerged in this process, an essential part of which was a feeling of inner resource and a growing awareness that, because of her inner flooding tendency, her life required special care and tending. She discovered that she could not afford to be too active and that meditative space in her life was essential. In this process, she thus learned how the shadow of her madness limited her, but also how this limitation was effective in bringing to birth an inner sense of and care for the self. As a result, psychic reality was born.

As this case progressed, levels of union began to emerge between us which included erotic fields, albeit marginally. To discuss this further I would like to detour from the case and reflect further upon issues of madness and sexuality in Jung's works.

Jung, Madness, and Sexuality

Aside from constraints on dealing with madness, another issue Jungian analysts have had to confront is the apparent lacunae in Jung's thoughts concerning sexuality and the body. In this context, one might reflect upon his early childhood experiences and wonder if this absence does not follow the dictates of repression.[4] But consider the following remarkable quote from his autobiography:

> In retrospect I can say that I alone logically pursued the two problems which most interested Freud: the problem of "archaic vestiges," and that of sexuality. It is a widespread error to imagine that I do not see the value of sexuality. On the contrary, it plays a large part in my psychology as an essential — though not the sole — expression of psychic wholeness. . . . The question of the chthonic spirit has occupied me ever since I delved into the world of alchemy. Basically, this interest was awakened by that early conversation with Freud, when, mystified, I felt how deeply stirred he was by the phenomenon of sexuality. (Jung 1961, p. 168)

Jung tells us, as part of the same quote, that his work on sexuality is found in "The Psychology of the Transference" and in *Mysterium Coniunctionis*.

In his alchemical studies, as these works exemplify, he takes sexuality either as a symbol of union or as a dangerous incestuous field to be transformed through the integration of projections. Aside from acknowledging sexuality on its own as a component of Dorn's *caleum* (1952, par. 702), that substance necessary for the union of mind and body, in his writings it largely remains either dangerous or a symbol that he employs in his quest to envisage the individuation process in alchemical symbolism. So what are we to make of Jung's assertion on the important role of sexuality in his psychology? He says that the "chthonic spirit" occupied him ever since he delved into alchemy, and that means for nearly forty years.

Jung's main point in his essay "The Psychology of the Transference" is, as I see it, that the union states achieved through these "lower waters" of the Anthropos (or of Dionysus as he refers to them in his analysis of the *Rosarium Philosophorum*) is on the same level of vitality and importance, if not identical to the spiritual union known as the *unio mystica* (1946b par. 418). But there is a major difference between the two: one can know the transcendent Self in an isolated way, as Jung knew the pleroma in his visions, but to discover the same phenomena through the *coniunctio* with another person, although partaking of the same energies, is a very different experience. Here personal and archetypal intertwine, yet the gap between them is ever present, save in moments of grace of their union. Suffering this gap that can never be crossed in the space–time life of the flesh without falling victim to the madness of inflation, often subtly concealed as it is, becomes a path to an experience of a container for the chthonic energies of the body. This sense of containment entails feeling a rhythm of container–contained between patient and analyst, for the patient is also a containing partner in this process. Within this interactive field one can experience a simultaneity of personal and archetypal, self and other, body and spirit.

Jung's alchemical studies — while indeed often avoiding and obscuring the importance of sexuality, the body, and embodiment — have nevertheless laid the path for the deeper exploration of this area. Where, we might ask, have Freud's heirs gone in this realm of sexuality and the body? Has psychoanalysis not avoided the body and sexuality as it has oriented to object relations, separate paths for drives and narcissistic libido, and the reduction of the manifestation of so-called preoedipal sexuality to either fusion needs or reactions to abandonment? But aside from the notable work of a few analysts, it seems to me that in psychoanalysis the erotic has been castrated and the body abandoned. Since Norman Brown's challenge in his book, *Life Against Death* (1959), the issue of the body has hardly been addressed, and Brown's project of going beyond sublimation and repression has never been taken up as a welter of clinical details of psychotic defense mechanisms have taken center stage.

If a union state occurs before mad parts have been acknowledged and lived with through submission to their power, it can be very dangerous. The danger, quite generally, is one of concretizing the interaction either in actual physical contact or else in a far too involved form of sharing which essentially denies that the analytic process is a special form of relationship that must, each session, be entered and exited. Instead, the process's effects linger for the patient, creating a very intense transference that readily becomes delusional. But if madness is first integrated, in this sense of knowing one's limits, then a union state often emerges with far less dangerous consequences, one that is experienced by both people as a "third thing" with important therapeutic results. In particular, this field acts like a container and a magnet that pulls in split-off aspects of psyche, notably the schizoid ego, which is the core sector of weakness that so terrifies everyone.

First and foremost, this fusion field, which is an important characteristic of our chthonic life, is a level of psyche in which the opposites are not separated. This means we do not experience them in projective identification but rather as a symbiotic state with a field quality that brings on a sense of unreality. This was the situation in the material presented above. I would like to now return to this case.

Clinical Material, Continued

Beneath our mutual attempts to find order in our encounter, there lurked the chthonian realities Paglia has spoken of, "the blind grinding of subterranean force, the long slow suck, the murk and ooze" (1990, p. 5f). And, as the patient said, "this muck was the madness that a powerfully idealized mother would protect me from experiencing."

What helped her begin to let go of her desire to be idealized and find an idealized object was a memory of a rare authentic moment she shared with her mother when she was about eighteen. After some discussion, her mother had not responded with her usual idealization and awe or devaluation and contempt, e.g., "I learn so much from you" or "You don't know the trees from the forest," but said with bewilderment and frustration, "You are like dry ice. I think I am going to touch something cold but it's hot instead." For the first time, she got feedback that conveyed the effect, albeit a frustrating one, that she had on another person. This was real to her, and, as in the episode of the article she'd written, it shows how a self, seeking the truth, was latent within her. In her sanest parts, it seemed a desire for the truth remained. Perhaps the difference between a good and poor prognosis in dealing with psychotic areas lies in this capacity.

Soon after the integration of her mad parts, the patient experienced the "presence" of the numinous on two separate occasions. Before she had only known this in a very abbreviated manner and in early childhood.

After I finished an earlier version of this paper, as I always do with clinical material, I showed what I had written to the patient. This initiated an important process. In showing her what I had written, I was somewhat anxious about her response, especially concerning its accuracy, but primarily I was enthusiastic about our work. She responded by expanding upon her material and, furthermore, offered her journal entries with permission to quote them as she felt was pertinent to the work we had done. Here is an example of such an entry:

> I stay home, resist being a "stimulus junkie," and hold on to giving myself time and space to linger. I meditate and after pause to look at the mountains.
>
> A numinous presence visits me. The presence is me. I am in a bed because I am very weak. It is not clear whether I am old or ill. A young adult couple — not sure exactly who they are — come to visit me. I feel very peaceful because they are not going to ask anything of me, and I won't ask anything of myself. I don't feel I have to give anything in my physical state. There is a connection to the Tao and not the more familiar feeling of dread.
>
> I feel my heart open to receiving their love. It means a lot to me that they came to visit me. I want to convey this — this comes up from me. There is a person at my side who knows me and reads my almost inaudible, incomprehensible utterances, much like the physicist Stephen Hawking's colleague understands his. It is almost comforting to have this person there. Instead I decide to communicate on my own. I use sign language and touch my heart. I am physically weak, but profoundly alive to deep emotion — deep love.
>
> This reminds me of a vision, the only one I ever had, when I was about five years old. (It was "out there," while what I have just described was not so separate, more like a lucid dream.) I wake up in the middle of the night and three women — three generations appear at the side of my bed. Their full build and full skirts remind me of Gypsies or the woman [Aunt Jemima] on the pancake box. They all have kerchiefs wrapped around their jaw and tied at their head, as if they all have toothaches. I am scared at first, but they don't

move. I am still frightened but less so. My fear lifts as the sun rises and it gets lighter and lighter until they disappear. They have been with me all my life.

I am struck that they cannot speak. I cannot speak in my recent vision. "My earliest claim to fame" according to my mother was that I was the earliest talker—people could not believe that a child of eleven months could talk so much and so well. I did not walk (as recorded in the same baby book) until I was fifteen months old.

A journal entry from a month later:

It is a little easier to resist the temptations to respond to some stimulus calling my name, and I again hold on to giving myself time to be.

I remember a convent my father would point out when we went on family car rides. Each time, in a ritualized way, he would say, "Those nuns behind the tall grey stone wall never see the light of day. They take a vow of silence and pray all day. No one looks in and no one looks out." On cue everyone in the car except me squealed and squealed at the thought. I quietly imagined a rectangular courtyard where I would be walking with the nuns in contemplative prayer.

Again a numinous presence visits me. It is a vibration, a rumbling and a revving that I feel in my whole body. It is very powerful and wants me to get going. A Hell's Angel moves his hands on my shoulders as if he is rotating the handlebars and is revving up his motorcycle. I realize this is what I have been up against my whole life and this Hell's Angel is too powerful, too forceful to go away. It is inside me.

Previously, like her madness, this had only been known to her as an outer force, like the Old Testament Yahweh. Now it, too, began to be part of the self that was growing as an inner psychic reality.

What then followed was remarkable. We had been working together for seven years and absolutely no elements of what I am about to describe had been present, but now there was an actual, palpable sense of linking between us that included, for both of us, an opening of the heart. This change led to the further embodiment of the Self structure that was achieved through integrating her mad parts. When the patient then felt these parts in her body, she became aware of the reality from which she had always been split, the truth that she had rarely ever been really present with me. She also felt how little, if any, container she had. Instead, she could now painfully experience how her ideas and feeling just spilled out and dissociated amidst moments, at best, of real contact. To finally feel this meant that she did now have a deeper sense of a containing self, but the real truth and power of this newly found state only came when she felt more embodied. That is, only when she breathed, relaxed her muscles, and allowed her feelings and affects free movement within her as she gave attention without interference to what these were or were about.

In this case, which is a relatively mild example, the patient was able to experience her madness without forming a strong psychotic transference. Often, this does not occur, especially with incest victims, who are usually deeply caught in the seemingly impossible symbiotic field as represented by Cybelle's possession of Attis.

The exploration of the psychotic part is an ongoing process in which one uncovers levels previously masked by defenses that had hidden them from any object's view. For example, in the case I have been discussing, the patient, on her own initiative, met with a colleague and suggested that I lecture at a conference the colleague was giving. After she told me this, I noted being pleased and interested but also felt somewhat disoriented and unconscious. As this state passed, I began to ask her to clarify something when she stopped me and, with great embarrassment, said that she knew she had to tell me that she was upset because I had not thanked her for what she had done. She felt very upset at noting she had these feelings. As I could reflect upon what I had experienced in my prior near abasement of consciousness, it was clear that I felt if I said nothing, I was acting as if we had a state of total communication between us, yet if I said something, it would have felt as if I was being formal and distancing with her. As I reflected in this way, it was immediately clear to me that these were not the only possibilities. I could have spoken to her in a heart-felt manner while I thanked her, and the state of distance and formality would not have occurred. Yet, while we were going through the experience that led to her remark on thanking me, I did not feel I had this option. Instead, only the split opposites of fusion and extreme distance seemed possible, a split pair that structured my consciousness for the time being with the result of a loss of energy and cohesiveness.

I mention this experience in some detail because I find it essential to discuss such a process with the patient. It mirrors the patient's own inner world and exhibits it to the patient, as it were, showing a state that the patient had never been able to expose to another person. In this case, she knew that the need for me to thank her was an awkward, paranoid reaction and stemmed from a part of her that was hidden during our interaction.

Prior to this interaction, the patient had been able to encounter her schizoid ego. This was a structure that she had rarely known consciously, as her life had been an endeavor to be competent. It then became apparent that the deadness that she felt in me and so frightened her was not only related to me but primarily to her mother's internal states of mind. Once she could begin to own her ego weakness,

I felt less deadened in my interactions with her. For it was her deep state of weakness that had this deadened quality but also, as an aspect of her mother, was accompanied in that object relation by a sense of cruelty. She thus has numerous reasons to fear her own schizoid level. It could destroy others and herself: internal and external worlds could vanish.

One frequently finds this type of splitting from schizoid elements, but when they manifest, they do so with their characteristic feeling of weakness. It is important for the analyst to witness this condition; it is very real for the patient and very humiliating. It takes considerable courage for the person not to enter a manic flight into competence. Staying with the schizoid part and its weakness is essential, otherwise the object world remains a dangerous place, for in this domain, love becomes a devouring hunger and the possibility for love ever to feel safe is minimal. The person can experience himself or herself here as an animal that, out of intense frustration, wants to destroy the object. The rage that exists is a terrible problem for the schizoid person, or for anyone whose schizoid sector is strong, for this rage, which is paranoid and behaves like a hair trigger at the slightest empathic failure of the object, can be very destructive to relationships. But if the analyst does not split away from seeing the patient's essential helplessness here, a transformative process can develop.

This drama is one that especially unfolds once idealizing defenses diminish. For the person, splitting from experiencing the schizoid level tends not only to idealize others defensively but also his or her own capacities. Once the state of weakness is experienced and owned, idealization and attendant inflation fades in its splitting strength, and a hungry rage can emerge.

When the patient revealed her need to be thanked, and we could establish the split opposites that existed in our interactive field, it was clear that we were experiencing the opposites in her psychotic part, but now they had a different form. Previously the opposites manifested as a split mirror, with each part demanding total control and adherence to its structure. In fact, when she felt her impulse to ask me to thank her and was embarrassed at this need, she tended to withdraw into a narcissistic shell, a protective bubble in which she needed no one. This type of defense existed previous to the discovery of her psychotic part. At that time, she defended against this part with a narcissistic bubblelike structure in which she played the roles of subject and object. At these times, I would feel odd, like an observer; she would be in a kind of rhapsody over her achievements, stating something she had done or

thought and then adoring herself for it in a way that felt a bit embarrassing to me because it was so extreme. But unlike the narcissistic
character, this was not her normal state. Rather, it emerged, I later
understood, when the pressure of her psychotic part was beginning to
force its intrusion into her conscious world. To protect against this, she,
in a sense, created her own form of madness which was a life in a
narcissistic bubble, cut off from the world that she idealized with the
same fervor with which she idealized herself. As this defense changed
and her psychotic part emerged, the mirrorlike quality of the opposites
in her psychotic part was the result of her narcissistic structure overlay-
ing these opposites. Now, as her deeper, schizoid issue manifested, the
opposites no longer emerged as a split mirror but now each had a
schizoid aspect, felt by me in a tendency to withdraw and become
enervated.

Exploration of a Mutual Field

This entire process and nearly all the words I have used to describe
it were told to the patient and also derived from our mutual discussion.
I must emphasize that this is an exploration of a mutual field, and
while I might at times speak of *her* ego weakness, I would only do so
after the patient has come to this understanding. Prior to this, I
embraced this weakness as a field quality which we both may possess.
All understandings were achieved through exploring the field, not as
my interpreting parts of her put into me, so to speak, in projective
identification. I never really knew, at the time, why I was feeling as I
did, for example, withdrawn, split, and unable to make good contact,
but allowing this state to exist and exploring it allowed each of us to
own what was ours and be enlivened by that connection.

Generally, these are archetypal dynamics. One can find this kind
of weakness, dismemberment, and attack in numerous myths. Egyptian myths are a storehouse of such imagery, as are various Dionysian
tales. The interactive field is structured by such imagery, and prematurely interpreting one's experiences in terms of projective identification can undermine the patient's capacity to own the fundamental
weakness and madness that has so disturbed, often in ever so subtle
fashion, his or her entire life. The analyst must really entertain the
possibility that the states of mind one experiences are one's own and
deal with them as such, even displaying them to the patient in a spirit
of exploration. This is a very different situation from using the patient
to deal with unmetabolized affects. Instead, one wrestles with affects

that can never be fully metabolized but, instead, must be respected for their overwhelming nature.

In this manner, we discovered how her schizoid ego was enmeshed in her psychotic part, and how severely distorting reactions could manifest within her, leading to tendencies to withdraw or narcissistically defend. Seeing this drama is what is essential. It is in our perception of this condition without judgment but instead with concern and without a need for the patient to be different, that the renewing potential within the archetypal level can become active. Just as, in Egyptian myth, Osiris's scattered parts are collected by Isis, and also as he does rise up out of his state of weakness, and as the persecutory anxieties represented by Seth are also tamed, so too the psychotic level can change and the schizoid ego can transform. It does not become a new solar hero, it always is weak and subject to being emotionally flooded, and withdrawal is always a potential, but it can become a structure with a sense of mystery and, strangely, a source of soul, a renewed inner life.

Let me briefly summarize the case to this point; what it further revealed was the strange logic in the psychotic part. First, we established the incommensurable opposites in her psychotic part. Then she recognized how the affect storms she had always suffered were really part of her, i.e., they ceased to have a transcendent quality for her, something "out there" that entered, and were instead felt as something within her psyche and on the edge of what she knew and experienced in herself. The psychotic part was not dealt with through interpretation, but rather required that I suffer its affects within an interactive field as part of the discovery of this sector in the patient. As a result of her awareness of this limiting sector, she and I began to experience our connection in a totally new way. For the first time, there was a sense of union between us, and further, there was a sense of a heart connection. We further discovered the layer of her schizoid ego and its humiliating sense of helplessness.

If someone is so defended against such madness as in the overwhelming affects this patient suffered and the peculiar splitting, confusion, and shame that she had to exclude from consciousness through excessive doing rather than being, then the possibility of a heart connection is nil. And if union states occur, they become so terrifying, often to both patient and therapist, as to result in splitting from emotional contact in a way that is terribly destructive to the patient. Only actual acting out is worse than this splitting by the therapist.

The Logic of the Psychotic Part

When we continued to explore her mad parts further and the field of madness between us, we discovered a peculiar kind of energy field within this sector. While the opposites were at first in a totally split state with each part vying for total control, now, when the split could be lived in, she could feel a different state. Rather than a total irreconcilable split, now a peculiar logic existed between these states. She would say that she didn't feel dead in this place, but neither did she feel alive. She did not feel empty, but neither did she feel full. A strange neither-nor logic pervaded this sector, a logic that could be perceived once the union state between us occurred and resultant states of madness could be further explored, in particular her deeply schizoid ego and its sense of energy loss and essential weakness. As part of the union process and its exploration, a growing together of the opposites began to take place. But the imagery that attended this state was grotesque. A dream (which is a good portrayal of the sector of her personality to which the analysis took her) exemplified this process:

Dream: *There is a supernatural event, cataclysmic. I am a passenger in a car and a man is driving. We are by the ocean. Nothing moves. The sand is solid but not cold or frozen. Footprints don't form. The ocean is still but I don't see that. The air is still, not sunny but not grey. School is closed. It is a weekday. Everything stopped. First the beach is empty, then it is not. There are groups of people, in black and grey dress, standing together, almost like sculptures. There is no sense of aliveness, yet no sense of death.*

I am in a building. A woman gives me four new boxes of crayons. They are all different colors. It is a wonderful surprise. There is a sense of hope and life.

I go to another room. A woman is there who scolds me for not being in the synagogue. I walk around and find a class of adolescent boys who are drawing. Their pictures have a black background and gold designs, drippings like a Jackson Pollock picture. They are wonderful. I pick up or have gold flakes, gold sparkles, and place them on a picture. The boys seem okay about that. I am aware that I didn't ask them. The pictures now look nicer both to me and to them. I give a glass jar holding the gold flakes to a boy and he sprinkles them on his picture. I think this class is so well behaved. I will leave a note for their teacher, a commendation note.

*I look for paper, but I can't find the right paper. I am then
confused about how to spell accommodation. I go back and forth
spelling commendation and then accommodation, getting terribly
confused. I write a note, I throw it away. It is from a brown piece
of paper bag. I cross out a word. The teacher in fact may have
passed by and I told him. But I am still focused on the note. I
stand back and am aware of how stuck I am and how crazy this is.*

The dream shows an entrance into a state of madness, symbolized
by the energy that is neither alive nor dead, into a place of life and
renewal, symbolized by the colors, and then to a place where she finds
gold that can transform blackness, and finds it amidst adolescent boys.
Then she is again in madness, this time caught between opposites of
commending someone or being accommodating, back and forth until
she herself realizes she is mad and is terribly exhausted.

What is exceptional here is that she cannot stay with the boys and
the gold. Why? The adolescent boys represent an energy of sex and
aggression that is extremely powerful. Dealing with this level proved to
be very slow and tenuous. Clearly, extremely engulfing energies lurked
here, and she was rightfully cautious about approaching them. At one
point, she told me that, in the meditations she had been doing for
several years, she found that breathing stopped at her belly and that
she felt a strong need for control here, as if she was using her will not to
fragment. To this point, this had been successful. After the dream
material of adolescence, however, her meditation became a source of
concern for her because she was beginning to fragment; her will was not
holding her together. For the first time, she wondered if she might
need medication. But by helping her to breathe differently, especially
showing her how to allow her breath to emerge from centers lower than
her belly and how to feel the exhalation as a wave moving down her
body through which her pelvic area relaxed, she found that her meditations improved and her fears of completely losing her mind were no
longer an issue.

I will leave this case at this point, hoping that it has helped to
clarify various configurations of the opposites in the psychotic part, the
peculiar logic latent in that area, the schizoid problem, and, most
essentially, the way a self can manifest out of accepting one's limitations
in the face of one's mad areas.

Summary

Madness and sexuality are often coupled. The reason for this, I believe, is that the erotic life of the body exists within a matrix of structures that contain so much energy, social prohibition, and, most important, the history of repression of those structures of religious life once associated with the religion of the Great Goddess, that the more deeply Eros is embraced, the more one enters near to those waters of madness, and conversely. It is these chaotic waters in which reality is distorted, the waters that the alchemists said were both a poison and a cure, that can lead to renewal and a new self structure, especially one that includes the body.

The solution to the problem of the destructive nature of the fusion state employed by patriarchal religion, and also by Jung in much of his writings, has always been a spiritual one, a quest for a spiritual Self that relieved the pain and bypassed the issue of the chthonic order.[6] This is a search for a self as container that defends against these energies, as if a place were carved out in a primal sea, outside of which these chaotic energies lived. Psychoanalytic tradition follows this path in its emphasis upon abstinence and awareness that sexuality in the transference can be a defense against deeper anxieties. Thus, the unobtainable erotic life of the body and the experience of being-in-the-body as a vehicle of spirit and imaginal life is treated as exactly that, forever lost to tangible and affective experience.

When we deal, in psychotherapy, with so-called preoedipal levels such as the Attis-Cybelle myth represent, we meet those "archaic structures of the mind" Jung referred to in his stated affinity with Freud's ideas, but, as in Jung's dissent from Freud's approach, the spiritual significance of sexuality becomes a burning issue. At this level, the analyst must really feel and suffer the loss of incestuous fulfillment; this is the true sacrifice of the animal life of the unconscious.

What is so difficult in the process of psychotherapy at this level is the paranoid quality of distrust one often meets. This focuses upon the belief that the analyst won't really feel the pain of loss, that he or she won't be genuinely involved and changed. The analyst must be especially embodied and authentic here; this demands far more involvement and suffering than dealing with the oedipal level. Often analysts will hide from this difficult level by treating the patient's distress as if an oedipal level were at issue and the analyst an involved but also quite separate parental figure. But such attitudes only reveal the analyst's aloofness or subtle splitting or need for power and will tend to constellate the patient's well-justified paranoia. For example, a person will fear being torn to pieces by the depths of despair and abandonment that he or she has to suffer both for themselves and for the therapist. The person will often not only hear what the therapist says but what isn't said, and a terrifying rush of paranoid ideas will fill the spaces between the therapist's sentences. Yet, there is also the fact that some patients, often highly gifted and intuitive people, with a special capacity for entering the sacred erotic depths of this level, also exist with very rigid defenses which create an impossible paranoid quality in the analysis, which is to say, for that particular analyst–patient relationship. Within the analysis the patient, when these levels are constellated, cannot forgive the analyst's errors. All is seen, again and again, through these errors and through major distortions of what the analyst has said. Other patients are able to reflect better, and when their psychotic parts are touched, they can integrate them and also split from them when necessary. In a sense, working through this level is like a fairy tale in which one has needs, gains help along the way, makes mistakes, and is tested to the utmost. This is true for both parties. In a sense, the question is how much failure can their process take. The process patient and analyst go through is the source of the psychic structure that must be acquired by both of them. But only the right mix of courage, spirit, and innate strength will do.

I conclude by returning to the case example of the woman who had begun to integrate her madness. On New Years Day, she spent some time, as she said, "visiting with her Self symbols" and described this as follows: "I sit quietly and imagine visiting the frail woman. Her head rests on the woman's lap, and I am struck that the hand that strokes my head is strong. I stay for a while and remember that I want to visit the Hell's Angel, too. Much to my surprise, he is sitting quietly in a chair watching. What a surprise! I recall that I came to treatment because I knew if my life continued the way it was going, there would be no surprises and I would be alive only to the degree that I could be surprised."

The mad parts of sane people are forever a source of surprise and fear for both the patient and analyst as they interact in a mutual field. Always dangerous, but always potentially healing, these fields continually confront us with the borders and limitations of what we know and who we are and cause us to reflect and reframe our attitudes of how we can be present over and over again. Without this level of madness, analytical work becomes dull and dangerously repetitive, tending to become a matter of technique and knowledge alone. As one becomes "older and wiser," one tends to *know about* psyche, rather than experience what one doesn't know. Madness seems to be our very best ally in restraining the dangerous and soulless tendency of knowledge used to shield from the shock of new experience.

Notes

1. I am indebted to the (unpublished) work of Ms. Cesia Goldfeld for the idea of a split mirror.

2. All features of psychotic process that Eigen describes in *The Psychotic Core* (1986), all can be felt in the countertransference when the psychotic part of the patient constellates.

3. I was to learn later that I was a powerfully idealized mother who would not attack her and who could heal the terrifying fusion experiences she had had with her actual mother. She recalled being lulled into reverie with her mother, only to be abruptly shocked by her mother's unpredictable change into a headlong rush to some compulsive task. It felt, she said, like being suddenly thrown against the wall. Such experiences, violations of transitional space, the damage to which Winnicott has so alerted us, left her vulnerable to overwhelming anxieties. The discovery of her painful history of fusion needs and their violation was only later to emerge; at this point of working with her mad parts, I was most aware of my disorientation and sense of unreality.

4. In his autobiography, Jung comments upon his early years, ages three to four, when he suffered from a severe regression. This was prompted by his parent's discord and his mother's hospitalization. "I was deeply troubled by my mother's being away. From then on, I always felt mistrustful when the word *love* was spoken. The feeling I associated with 'woman' was for a long time that of innate unreliability" (1961, p. 8). During her absence, Jung recalls with an unusual and touching candor his erotic and loving feelings for a woman who cared for him. He also tells us that she was his first anima image. It causes one to wonder if the oedipal feelings he could not attach to his mother did thrive with this other woman and if, upon his mother's return, his only avenue was regression characterized by death wishes and an invasion by anal and oral fantasies. His anxieties became paranoid. The fragile character of repression for the young, three- to four-year-old child failed, as did his splitting defenses. His good objects became swallowed up; "Lord Jesus," at one time a comforting inner object, lost "the aspect of a big, comforting, benevolent bird and became associated with the gloomy black men in frock coats, top hats, and shiny black boots who busied themselves with the black box [in the graveyard]" (ibid, p. 10).

The young Jung's regression continued and culminated in his "first conscious trauma," seeing a person approaching and becoming "overcome with fear, which rapidly grew into deadly terror as the frightful recognition shot through my mind: 'That is a Jesuit'. . . . Probably he had evil intentions. . . . For days afterward the hellish fright clung to my limbs and kept me in the house" (ibid., p. 10f).

It is then remarkable to read Jung saying that from these early experiences his intellectual life is born (ibid., p. 15). He sought their meaning, as if his suffering was necessary to "bring the greatest possible amount of light into (his) darkness" (ibid.). Apparently, considering the enigma that his mother always remained for him, his early sexual issues were never returned to. Instead, they were spiritualized into an intellectual life.

5. If the Attis-Cybelle myth is any guide, humankind suffered a psychotic episode at the end of the Neolithic, and out of this psychosis solar rational thinking gradually emerged and totally suppressed the other kind of thinking and other relationship to the numinosum. Furthermore, we are still reeling from this psychotic episode. The dark, devouring face of the Great Goddess, Cybelle's madness, still haunts us, as it did the Latin poet Catullus in the first

century B.C. The last stanza of one of his poems (Number 63, in *The Poems of Catullus*) reads:

> Mighty Goddess, Goddess Cybelle, sacred Mistress of Dindymus,
> grant that my house may be kept safe from all of your furor, my Lady:
> Drive others off into frenzy, drive others into madness.

In the Attis myths, we also learn that when he attempted to find another lover in a nymph, Cybelle killed her. Out of his grief, he killed himself.

6. Jung's analysis of myths, for example, in *Symbols of Transformation*, considers them to represent deep, unconscious movements of psychic energy. The ego becomes aware of these energy transformations, for example, those represented by the motif of sacrifice, "in much the same way as sailors are made aware of a volcanic upheaval under the sea" (Jung 1952, par. 669). But myths, like dreams, are also often remarkably detailed replays of history, using metaphor to represent events of both actual and fantasy nature. When dreams can be perceived to have this quality, and one discovers the one-to-one fit between dream imagery and the previous day's events, the dream then has a purpose very different from seeing it as a symbolic statement. Instead, with the dream-as-metaphor, one can, as it were, see and remember oneself from the previous day, but now do so while in the body, as against the more mental and disembodied state for which the dream compensates. Dreams can function to bring the mental ego down into the body and thus into the truth, just as myths can function to remind a culture of the truth of its origins in a way that has a here-and-now significance.

Jung's approach to the Attis-Cybelle myth follows his libido theory. The castration of Attis thus represents the sacrifice of instinctual feelings that would regressively cling to the Great Mother. These feelings are represented by the animal that must be sacrificed, the animal in us "which fights with all his instinctive conservatism" against the individuation urge (Jung 1952, par. 653). For Jung, castration, as in the acts of the priests of Cybelle or in the image of the feeling of a pine tree, signifies the sacrifice of the libido, both as the incestuous love of the son for the mother and of her incestuous love for him (ibid.).

Jung also tells us that the impulse to sacrifice comes from the mother herself, who drives Attis to madness and self-mutilation. Thus, he further reasons, the impulse to sacrifice comes from the unconscious, for regression is inimical to life (Jung 1952, par. 660). He then adduces parallel themes, especially similarities between the Attis-Cybelle myth and the bull sacrifice in Mithraism. Mithra, he says, sacrifices the bull "willingly and unwillingly at once, hence the rather pathetic expression on certain monuments of Mithra" (ibid., par. 665). Jung quotes Cumont's description of Mithra during the sacrifice as follows: the head is slightly tilted backwards, so that his glance is directed towards the heavens, and the contraction of the brows and lips gives a strange expression of sorrow to the face (ibid., par. 666). But Jung then gives this his own twist when he says that "this facial expression represents sentimentality which is sister to brutality. . . . The morbid facial expression points to the disunity and split-mindedness of the sacrificer: he wants to and he doesn't want to" (ibid., par. 668).

But the pained expression on Mithra's face represents the suffering and loss of something beautiful and precious. The "contraction of the brows and lips gives a strange expression of sorrow to the face" because he is giving up one kind of relationship to the *numinosum* for another. Mithra gives up the energies known in the *hieros gamos* so that another avenue of development can occur, that achieved finally in the *unio mystica*. Later, in alchemy, these "older" energies return, and with them returns the very difficult task of relating to them without fusing by creating a different kind of body and a new sense of relating through subtle-body fields.

Jung's reading of history is that this kind of relation to the *numinosum* had to be sacrificed. In much recent literature, it is cast in the notion of a goddess cult that was overthrown at the end of Neolithic times by patriarchy or some such representation of a new form of male values. Jung would insist that this sacrifice was necessary, and his choice example is Christ's sacrifice in which not only is instinctuality sacrificed, "but the entire natural man" (1952, par. 673). This, Jung says, leads to the danger of consciousness being separated from its instinctual foundations and of setting up the conscious will in the place of natural impulse (ibid., par. 673). But only through this sacrifice "will the dominating idea of consciousness be in a position to assert itself completely and mould human nature as it wishes. . . . The attempt must be made to climb these heights, for without such an undertaking it could never be proved that this bold and violent experiment in self-transformation is possible at all" (ibid., par. 674).

This experiment, as Jung calls it, has had an ambivalent result at best. Mithra looks back upon his sacrifice with appropriate mourning, and Cybelle's madness and Attis's castration is much more than a representation of the transformation of the libido. It is a metaphorical replay of history at the end of the Neolithic period to which Cybelle dates. It is a replay of the inner experiences of people to a violent change in values, to a change that focused in a solar rational way.

References

Borgeaud, P. 1988. *The Cult of Pan in Ancient Greece*. Chicago: University of Chicago Press.

Brown, Norman. 1959. *Life Against Death*. New York: Norton.

Burkert, Walter. 1987. *Ancient Mystery Cults*. Cambridge, Mass.: Harvard University Press.

Catullus, n.d. *The Poems of Catullus*. Charles Martin, trans. Baltimore: Johns Hopkins Press, 1990.

Dehing, Jeff. 1990. Jung and knowledge: From gnosis to praxis. *Journal of Analytical Psychology*, 35, 2:193–211.

Detienne, M. 1989. *Dionysos at Large*. Cambridge, Mass.: Harvard University Press.

Eigen, M. 1986. *The Psychotic Core*. New York: Jason Aronson.

Goldfeld, Cesia. Private communication.

Grotstein, J. 1990. Nothingness, meaninglessness, chaos, and the "black hole." *Journal of Contemporary Psychoanalysis* 26, 2, 3; 27, 1.

Hillman, J. 1972. *The Myth of Analysis*. New York: Harper.

Joseph, S. M. 1987. Fetish, sign and symbol through the looking glass: A Jungian critique of Jacques Lacan's *Ecrits*. *San Francisco Jung Institute Library Journal* 7, 21.

Jung, C. G. 1946a. On the nature of the psyche. In *Collected Works* 8:159–234. Princeton, N.J.: Princeton University Press, 1960.

_____. 1946b. The psychology of the transference. In *Collected Works* 16:163–326. Princeton, N.J.: Princeton University Press, 1954.

_____. 1952. *Mysterium Coniunctionis. Collected Works,* vol. 14. Princeton, N.J.: Princeton University Press, 1963.

_____. 1952. *Symbols of Transformation. Collected Works,* vol. 5. Princeton, N.J.: Princeton University Press, 1956.

_____. 1961. *Memories, Dreams, Reflections*. A. Jaffe, ed. New York: Pantheon.

Kerenyi, C. 1976. *Dionysos*. Princeton, N.J. : Princeton University Press.

Lacan, J. 1977. *Ecrits*. A. Sheridan, trans. New York: Norton.

Otto, W. 1965. *Dionysos: Myth and Cult*. R. Palmer, trans. Bloomington, Ind.: Indiana University Press.

Paglia, Camille. 1990. *Sexual Personae*. New Haven, Conn.: Yale University Press.

Schwartz-Salant, N. 1989. *The Borderline Personality: Vision and Healing*. Wilmette, Ill.: Chiron Publications.

Searles, H. 1965. Transference psychosis. In *Collected Papers on Schizophrenia and Related Subjects*. New York: International Universities Press.

Notes on the Counterpart

Michael Eigen

Overview

What a burgeoning literature there is on the "counterpart." From its inception, depth psychology has been fascinated with the multiplicity of the self. Freud informally wrote of the unconscious as another kind of consciousness. His structural theory charts the interweaving of systems of otherness within the personality. Jung amplified this vision by describing an archipelago of encounters with the otherness of self, linked by growth of a true self thread. For Lacan, the unconscious is Other, made up of multiple Others, another place or scene, another language.

Winnicott's false self is a counterpart of true self. It may protect the true self, or act as a substitute, a counterfeit. False self is a reactive, defensive system. True self is the active center of personality. True self is allied with undefensive being, out of which creative doing grows. True self impulses grow out of open being. Pulsations of the true self often seem mad, tyrannical, or fearful, as well as inspiring, while a healthy false self may make life more fun, effective, and sane. Some people, like Van Gogh, live solely from true self feeling (see Winnicott on Van

Michael Eigen is associate clinical professor at the New York University Postdoctoral Program in Psychoanalysis and senior member, faculty training and control analyst at the National Psychological Association for Psychoanalysis in New York. His previous publications include *The Psychotic Core, Coming Through the Whirlwind*, and the forthcoming *The Electrified Tightrope: Between Catastrophe and Faith*.

Gogh, in Rodman 1987, p. 124). Too great an intolerance of false self or false self deficiency can be disastrous. Sometimes it is hard to tell the difference between true and false self and sometimes the distance between them is unbridgeable.

French authors have used "crypt" or "vault" to describe a sealed-off aspect of personality. More recently, Bollas (1989) used the term "ghostline personality." Such attempts portray dead counterparts.

I would like to organize my discussion of the otherness of the self around three main themes: (1) the taint; (2) the split; and (3) the "force" or nullity.

The Taint

Smith frequently described himself as tainted. The taint ran through his personality, his being. He felt this from his earliest days. He was a very alive and energetic man and lived a full life. He did a lot of true self living. Yet he felt the fabric of his life was warped: his true self was warped. He was a gay psychoanalyst who had affairs with young men. At the same time, he remained married to one woman throughout his adult life and had grown children, one of them a homeless schizophrenic.

When I saw Smith, he was a nearly broken man suffering from advanced heart disease. He sought help because one of his affairs threatened to ruin his professional career. It appeared the skew in his self had taken a cumulative toll.

What was true self, what false? Smith kept up a front with his family, yet had true affectional ties with his wife and children. He loved music. He was at once controlling, assertive, manipulative, and seductive, a charming man. At professional meetings, his remarks were discerning, probing, and open. He was sensitive to the most alive currents in the field. In his homosexual affairs, he lived out dramas around what Khan (1979, pp. 12–16) described as "the idolized self," a kind of manic, megalomanic binging on ideal feelings. At such moments, he felt most alive, but out of the corner of an eye he stared at the warp. The warp never left him. (I have written about Smith before in *The Psychotic Core* (1986, pp. 186–189) and "On Demonized Aspects of the Self" (1984).)

Poets write of a worm that spoils the rose of experiencing. Religions depict a tendency to spoil integrity or goodness. The Jewish bible erects a bulwark against the spoiling tendency, a system to manage the evil inclination, but difficulties proliferate. What violence love of Jesus unleashed upon the world! Psychoanalysis explores links between ideal and violent feelings and joins the sensitive thread in history of those who unmask lies we live.

Weil's (1958) "repressed bad self," a "garbage" or "shit self," Balint's (1968) "basic fault," especially the abysses of the "malignant regression," Bion's (1970) evocation of a poisoned self, a self not simply poisoned by a bad breast, but by the lie one lives: so many ways to circle in on the "off point," the skew, the warp, the wound that never heals.

The Split

The taint is often organized and expressed by splitting processes. In Smith's case, splitting was highly complex and dangerous. An observing mental ego never stopped working and oscillated between several attitudes. At times it was a befuddled onlooker, as if stupefied by events. Consciousness ticked like a clock but did not make sense of anything. Smith's life might have been lived by someone else, except, by an accident of fate, it happened to be happening to him.

By degrees a bemused smile would appear on the face of consciousness, a dapper devil, a sickly transcendence, the mockery of the victim victor, the eternal "heh-heh." Below the smile was the mute explosive body, really a body self: a screaming self, an exploding heart, or perhaps a heart that failed to explode but withered.

Ideal feelings blew in and out, lighting the whole system, leaving it in darkness. At times, the ideal filled Smith's eyes: a young man appeared who looked like perfection. At times, an eye-heart connection was made, and Smith courted his beloved as in a dream. More rarely still, a blessed moment of eye-heart-genital connection arose, which, as likely as not, would be spoiled by something. At times, the spoiler was an acute pang of hate, or doubt, or too zealous possessiveness. At times, painful differences obtruded as fusion mounted, or revulsion and unsatiated demand soiled the aftermath.

Smith might try to rev up the ideal feeling: if only it would last long enough to see an experience through. He could coast on it for a time, but effort was needed to keep it going. His realistic eye never stopped seeing. No fault escaped him, not his own, nor his lover's, but as long as the ideal feeling lasted, faults were irrelevant, even funny and endearing.

When "normal" ego functioning returned, Smith's efforts went into repairing the damage. He picked youths he could nurse. They fell apart and he took care of them. His mental or transcendental ego became parental, while body ego fragility and fragmentation was experienced through his lovers. He sometimes devoted years to efforts of rehabilitation and tended to be successful. Launching someone's life gave him great satisfaction. Smith bulled past intimations of his own weakness and felt strong and good as the helper. His life was encompassed by a sense of goodness. An inner factory incessantly turned bad feelings into good ones. Yet success was cloying. The warp never left. The taste of the warp pervaded the goodness. His body could not support the life his psyche fabricated and eventually collapsed beneath him.

In my books and papers I explore aspects of a split between an occultly transcendent mental self and a fusional-explosive body self. I take this split to be the core pathological structure of our time. The mental self may use knowledge of the world to navigate portions of life relevant to it. It may rely on cognitive maps, instrumental learning (means-end or causal relationships), and interpersonal observation. However, the mental self is more or other than scientist, philosopher, and political strategist. It is plugged into the "ideal" as well as "real."

Psychic systems carve themselves out of an ocean of ideal feeling. Megalomania is more than inflation. It is a reminder of the more from which we come. Deflation is as much a disease as inflation. The operational personality overly relies on means-end know-how and denudes life of fantasy. The smaller self fears losing territory to the larger self, and the larger self fears squeezing into restrictions and boundaries the smaller self takes for granted. Which is more afraid of which? (My book, *Coming Through the Whirlwind* (1991), includes dialogues between smaller and larger aspects of self, as an attempt to heal the split between them.)

Ideal feeling may take the form of omniscience in the mental self, omnipotence in the body self (Eigen 1986, Chapter 8). Omniscience-omnipotence often fills gaps where one might sense deficit. Coming up against deficit opens glimpses of underlying streams of ideal feeling held at bay by acts of knowing. The complexity of relationships between terms of experience may prompt us to side with one term against another (splitting), rather than stay alive to the play of similarity–difference. We are engaged in a long-term learning process, thousands of years old, in which we dimly apprehend workings of the diverse capacities that make us up and carry us along. Our destiny is to become partners with our capacities.

At times, it seems that ideal feeling becomes tainted and distributes itself along mental self/body self axes in poisonous ways. To an extent, splitting activities try to contain the taint. Klein (1946) and Fairbairn (1954) describe ways that selective dissociations save pockets of health from destructive absorption. We know only too keenly how containing structures become tainted and become part of the problem. We are always part of the problem, since we are figures in larger structures.

The Force: Adventures in Nullity

Bion wrote of "a force that continues after . . . it destroys existence, time and space" (1965, p. 101). After everything is destroyed, the force continues destroying. Destruction goes on in subzero dimensions. The existence of such a force is, perhaps, impossible, since it cancels existence, but that is precisely its power. Dante's Hell is amateurish next to regions of nullity evoked here.

The false self slows the force down. It variably absorbs, deflects, or binds fringes of the force. The false self can also further the work of the force. At such times it appears to be an offshoot, a ray of the force, driving the self deeper into nullity. More often, I believe, the false self is on the side of life. It expresses a refusal to die out or give up. It may protect the true self like a bad big brother. True self elements are usually mixed up in it.

The mix-up of true self/false self may hopelessly confuse a person. The force feeds on and takes advantage of this confusion to infiltrate the personality, so as to annihilate not only the true self but false self as well. Usually we worry about desecration of the true self, the holy spark within. We battle with compromises and lies that poison as they save us. Yet the false self has its own brand of holiness, as it tricks and wheedles and perseveres (like Jacob and Rebecca) to carve out a place where the best in us comes out. It refuses to forfeit the Blessing.

The force's conquest of true self appears to be relatively easier than conquest of false self. The force turns the energy of personality against itself (aggression against libido transforms into destructions of libido as companion to destruction of personality by libidinal flooding) and uses evidence of corruptibility to solidify despair (the conviction, hypnotic suggestion, or hallucination that integrity is lost forever and life is not worth living). At this point, it seems that the force is content with turning the false self into a devil (systems of devils) that persecutes, rather than protects, true self elements. The latter collapse under pressure as morale is undermined by bullying, cajoling, and propagandizing. The force promises the false self that it will lose nothing and gain everything: it will get more of what it wants and grow stronger (opportunistically and via long-range planning).

Taking advantage of enticements or opportunities can now be used as evidence of underlying weakness, a succumbing of true self elements. What is noble in the self hates itself. The false self capitalizes on the true self's grief by converting the latter's hatred of its corruptibility to hatred of weakness as such. False self feeds on true self weakness and traduces and recruits true self elements (it uses the latter to justify itself, if shame still exists in the scheme of things). The false self gloats at the true self's shame, provoking the true self to hide or disappear (go to another world) or seek the false self's protection. The force uses the false self to block or spoil the true self's connection with God (destruction of dependence as opening). True self hopes against hope that false self will save it, converting dependence to parasitic addiction (idolatry), as it plunges toward idiocy.

The bloated false self exploits true self's crises of faith. As long as there are crises there is agony, the personality's fever. What a relief to give in to false self and feel "peace" for a time. True self "learns" that its connection with God is too weak to save it: for all things that count in life, its connection with God is simply irrelevant. False self does so much more for it, so much more quickly. True self buries itself in false self's energy, and for a time life may go on better than ever.

True self's fearful clinging gives false self the illusion of indispensability. At the height of its power, false self ignores its sense that the force is using it. It is too caught up in its own momentum to care. Yet once true self has shifted its center of gravity from God to false self, the latter's work is over. The force dismantles and destroys it.

That the force goes on working after it destroys existence, time, and space, means that it destroys the various counterparts of existence, time, and space (Bion 1965, pp. 110–112). The false self is a privileged system of counterparts or substitutes. False self does not realize that victory weakens it. By absorbing true self, it cuts itself off from the larger destiny of existence. By weakening or nullifying true self's connection with God, false self loses support of its own ground. Head and gut split off and heart spins into oblivion or sentimentality.

Bion partly represents this state of affairs by putting existence and related terms in quotes. The force may be represented and

personified by a non-existent "person" whose hatred and envy is such that "it" is determined to remove and destroy every scrap of "existence" from any object which might be considered to "have" any existence to remove. Such a nonexistent object can be so terrifying that its "existence" is denied, leaving only the "place where it was." This does not solve the problem because the place where it was, the no-thing, is even more terrifying because it has, as it were, been further denied existence instead of being allowed to glut itself with any existence it has been able enviously to find. Denial of the existence of the "place where it was" only makes matters worse because now the "point," marking the position of the no-thing, cannot be located. (Bion 1965, pp. 111–112)

Bion's conclusion (probably starting point) is that the force may be anywhere. We reach a world of horrific boundlessness in relation to which the term *nameless dread* seems strangely small. If God is a circle whose center is everywhere and circumference nowhere, the force is the counterpart whose center is a vortex or black hole (anywhere and everywhere) which is determined that no part of God or God's creation will escape it.

Bion gives figurative form to this horrific formlessness by personifying it as *a nonexistent "person."* It is hard not to think of Milton's Satan with his yawning abysses and formless infinite and darkness visible and palpable. But it is far too easy to transform Satan into a dashing adventurer, swashbuckling and appealing (romantic vitality), a sophisticated and debonair gentleman (ironic) or entertainer (cynical), an efficient engineer, businessman, or entrepreneur. None of these images are derealized or depersonalized enough. They are bits of wish fulfillments, promises. Such devils are too lively to circumscribe the realms at stake here. A therapist might be quite happy if a patient who is *a nonexistent "person"* should be lucky enough to fall into the hands of such a devil and risk a breakthrough into life.

It is clinically important to see shades of unreality. In Bion's description, "person" is in quotes, nonexistent is not in quotes. Here, nonexistence is real: the force is real. "Person" has become a cipher, a "place" where a person was, a person manqué, an "as if" personality. Let us assume that the force has already devoured the person or the realness of the person. Now it devours the unperson or unrealness of the nonperson. It devours the shell that is left, the counterpart of the person, the empty phony version, the dead false self. The dead false self is an impostor or proxy of the lively false self. Our Bionic Virgil leads us through worlds of counterpart systems, region after region of nullity.

If the therapist directs his remarks to the person, when the person has vacated to region after region of nonperson, his efforts are likely to be appropriated by fringes of a dead false self system and shuttled toward the vortex to disappear. It may be that elements of the therapist's communication and true self elements of the patient find each other, whether in the vortex, dead false self, live false self, or in God. Such finding is always possible: it is never too late. But life calling to life does not nullify the helpless paralysis in which life is stuck: it may seem too late when living is more horrible than dying.

Much depends on the therapist's range finder. If, by a stroke of luck, genius, or hard work, he hits the right shade at the right time, something may happen. Usually the shade will shake it off: disturbance is taboo. Freud's depiction of a system that aims to reduce stimulation to zero is an example of a range finder that scores a hit. We observe shades zeroing the struggle to communicate. The person does not appear to have a chance. Nevertheless, a shade occasionally shakes off the mist, and instead of only an agonized groan and the fall back to zomboid oblivion, a creaky, pained smile of recognition reaches out with bony fingers, remnants of a bashful ecstasy. Dry bones, indeed! So much of the problem is that ecstasy has no place to go, and the force channels it.

Smith's Dissolution: Peace at Last

Throughout most of his life, Smith maintained or lived off a live false self. Enough true self elements found recognition through the live false self to make live worth living. His sexual and reparative activity, musical interests, psychoanalytic work, involvement with his family: all enhanced his sense of aliveness. Yet he felt a thread of falseness running through the activities he valued most. Even his most intense sexual moments felt "tainted" (Smith's term). He *knew* he was a superior psychoanalyst but did not let intimations of his autocratic and manipulative use of patients slow him down. He *knew* he was a good father and husband and glossed over his hand in his wife's and children's difficulties.

Smith had a hardened and impenetrable view of the objectivity of life's events, including characterological makeup. He did not accept responsibility for his children's madness. They had their own lives to live, as did he. We all march to our own drummers, have our own timetables. His wife chose him, and he chose her: they were responsible for their choices. Their lives would have been shallower and poorer without each other. In his own way, he was devoted to his family: he *stayed* with them. He was proud of his steadiness, his staying power. He lasted the course. He stayed with his profession as well. He saw it through. He played down his awareness of how controlling and emotionally detached he had been. If he had regrets or self-recriminations, they were consigned to oblivion. He pointed to the good he had done, and he had done much good. He used his analytic training to maintain a balanced view of things, tipped in his favor.

Smith could not let down. Even when he finally wept, he did not let down so much as let things out. Rage toward the mother with whom he identified poured out. She was the strong, mad boss who teased him with the chickens she decapitated. His father caved in and killed himself when Smith was five. Letting down was more than dangerous: it was deadly. He was aware of becoming a version of his mother, not only to survive, but to be empowered. He feared and hated her but sympathized with her, too. She saw the family through. Without her crazy strength, life would have crushed them. Her power that was part of him enabled Smith to lift himself out of poor, deprived surroundings and make something of himself.

Smith remained plugged into her mad strength all his life. He lost contact with his fear and weakness. He was rightfully proud of how far he had come. He scarcely believed it. Who would have believed his rise from southern rural poverty to big city success? In his estimation, he had "made it." He had done it by himself but could not have done it without the vitality he felt from her. He was trapped by her strength.

Why did Smith come to see *me*? He was nearly twenty years my senior and more highly positioned. I seemed frightened and weak next to him. Perhaps he thought he could rehabilitate me like the youths he took over. Yet come he did, and he persisted until his death.

We had seen each other at professional meetings and had been in a peer study together. I was surprised to learn that he had listened carefully to my remarks. He felt he could count on me to speak truth and hear him out. I thought I had been on the quiet side in the peer group, although I got into arguments. Smith felt I honestly tuned into things. He felt he could be free with me. I gradually learned that he also saw in me a strength that came through suffering. Nevertheless, next to Smith I could not help but feel I was to hold the place where fear and weakness might have been, and often I was fear itself.

I don't think I ever quite exuded the self-confidence and ease Smith did. My self-esteem seemed low next to his. Perhaps he hoped to play the phallic idol to my admiring self, but the transference did not quite take this turn. He was so identified with the saving maternal aggressor that it seemed my job to speak truth for the child that got left behind: the child that became a no-thing.

His personality seemed eaten by a secret battle to be something rather than nothing. His life was marked by fierce struggle, and his pleasure in professional competence, love of music, and sexual ecstasies provided some relief. Without work and music, life would have been hell. Sexuality led him into tormenting, dangerous situations. He tried to make family life a haven, but it was filled with pain and failure. His wife and children accused him of trying to fob them off with a shell of himself, although he had given them whatever he could. Worst of all, Smith related to his secret pain as something to handle, as if expertise could deal with it and somehow nullify it.

He did not expect *me* to nullify it, but *he* chronically did so. Smith was the psychoanalyst who understood the origins of his difficulties. He knew all the why's. He rode above his feelings as fast as he bared them. He could not simply suffer and cry and say how awful it all was. He always had to be doing something to it, to understand it, turn it this way and that, to stay on top of it.

For a time, I suspected Smith of using me to keep his job. I wrote all the needed letters confirming that he was working on his problems, that the work place need not fear him. As usual, the threat of disaster abated. The young man who had accused him visited Smith in the hospital after a heart attack and dropped the charges. Smith said the young man's family was grateful to him for guidance he gave. Smith always managed to get out of things.

But he could not stop his body clock. I felt more at ease after the crises with work passed, and Smith continued working. It did not occur to me that he had come to therapy to die. He seemed to be battling for life. To me, Smith seemed to push past himself, not get low enough to connect with himself. To me, it seemed that a chronic false self style had become his real self. But Smith kept saying that he was getting closer to himself, that he had never come this close. He said that, at last, he was getting to his center. He felt a peace that had eluded him. Only in retrospect do I see that Smith linked up with himself before he died. It was a praiseworthy feat, because he did it through layers of ego coverings that never left.

Now I wonder if Smith didn't choose me precisely because I was offbeat, not in the mainstream. His maverick qualities hid under a far more conventional bearing. He tied things up more than I. I was more loose ends. It was precisely my quirkiness he valued. I must have reminded him of himself, an alternate self, a counterpart. We shared an ironic sincerity, a sense of devotion. We both had a cynical, mocking side, but mine was tempered by faith, his by ego control. Faith is the center. I wonder if this aspect of the devotion to which he resonated was what attracted him.

Perhaps I was a proxy for the outsider he left behind, but also a caring, mischievous child. In some ways, my lack of development worked for me. Smith's stronger, more sophisticated ego placed too much strain on his body. I could not hold on to myself as long as he seemed to be able to hold on to himself. He was able to maintain a sort of psychoanalytic consciousness far more rigorously, incessantly than I. I dropped into dumb being more readily and completely than he and had to rouse myself to think something, whereas he was always thinking. He was always controlling trauma by psychoanalytic thinking. Sometimes he made my head spin in sessions and I had to shut off.

I never scored a hit when I referred to diffusion or fragmentation, but I can't help feeling that the wholeness Smith felt listening to music (especially Gustav Mahler) was, partly, a measure of absent dispersal. Also, his liking me in my awkward intensity, his acceptance of me when I was ill at ease, surely this must have been some kind of mirror. I well understand how he helped people. Yet he was not only smooth, nor I only awkward. There was an earthy aspect to his sophistication, and I was far from naive.

What I now see, through our defensive layerings and differing styles, is soul smiling at soul. Soul recognizing soul. This is what we felt when we exchanged glances at meetings or felt warmly toward each other across a room. I would not say we were soul brothers or partners, but there was some kind of kinship. It is not enough to say we both knew hell: not all hells get along together. Perhaps it was where our souls open to heaven that most attracted Smith. Our therapy was not only about missing fear and weakness. Together we created/discovered a place where ecstatic longing could not be x'd out by psychoanalytic consciousness (or a narrow form of the latter).

The path was not through diffusion but emptiness. Smith did not let down but began to speak of emptiness. It is hard to convey how miraculous this felt. What an emptiness ran through the fullness of his personality! What emptiness he gave vent to! He spoke of a bottomless, inexhaustible emptiness: a painful, agonizing emptiness. The fullness of living did not stop because of this emptiness. The fullness of living kept right on going; it had its own power and momentum. But emptiness was everywhere, in the fullness, too. This was the closest Smith came to losing ego control, with the exception of the first panicky moments of therapy when he feared the loss of his university position.

In those first visits, I felt that Smith's personality was disintegrating, but he pulled out of it like a skilled pilot. I suspect finding a place to deposit himself (psychoanalysis) enabled the nose dive to stop and controls to return. It was only through the emptiness of his controls that Smith could contact himself. The gradient of the psychoanalysis was toward this emptiness, although neither he nor I could know this. To me, it seemed Smith's contact with himself was several times removed, but it felt otherwise to him. Emptiness wiped out distance: he felt the pain directly.

The painful emptiness stayed with Smith, and he with it, for nearly half a year. Through it he began to feel ecstasy. The ecstasy did not nullify the emptiness, not any more than the emptiness nullified the fullness of living. These currents went on together, sometimes more, sometimes less distinguishable. It seems accurate to say that when the intensity of emptiness peaked, another dimension or world of experiencing opened.

Smith's ecstasy was not what one might call a cosmic ecstasy but a psychoanalytic ecstasy. His smaller psychoanalytic "why" consciousness, addicted to causal visions and explanations, continued ticking. But now the illusion of control this gave him seemed less important than the moment of experiencing. He began to dip into his emotional currents a bit more like the way he listened to music. The emphasis was less on the power of understanding than on emotional impact and appreciation. His love for psychoanalysis reached a new place.

Most of his adult life Smith used psychoanalysis to maintain his equilibrium and enhance his self-esteem. It functioned as a kind of psychic cooling system. Now it became a tool to heat things up. Smith now clung to psychoanalysis as a vehicle for heightening experiencing, rather than as a weapon of pseudomastery.

Psychoanalytic thinking was the thread that knit his life together. What would have become of him without it? It was not just his formal analyses that were important, but the whole psychoanalytic milieu: readings, meetings, colleagues, a total way of life. The psychoanalytic insights that popped into his head were supported by an entire community from which he drew nourishment. Friends, enemies, critics, admired and despised protagonists: through psychoanalysis he found a *world*, a place.

Now he found much more. Psychoanalysis was becoming what he always hoped it might be: a way to face himself, to open himself. It was in relationship to psychoanalysis that Smith came closest to an act of repentance and atonement. He felt grateful for psychoanalysis because it had given him a life. For the first time he not only *saw* but *faced* misuse of his lover (psychoanalysis was his true love). He had used psychoanalysis to close wounds, not to open his heart. At last, psychoanalysis shined as an opening of self. What peace this lacerating moment brought!

"I don't want to lie now," said Smith. "It's important not to. I can't stand lying anymore. This is the first time I'm not bullshitting myself. I must get to things as they are. I've got to." Smith called to himself through his shells with an urgency that shattered lies. Can anyone stop lying? Wouldn't total lack of self-deception be inhuman? Perhaps only the devil, father of lies, is totally honest. Yet Smith *had* to break through to himself.

Apparently Smith knew something I didn't. I now see that he sensed death was imminent, that he was in a now-or-never situation. He kept up a good front to the end (after hospital stays, he continued his psychoanalytic practice). I know he valued his work with me. He repeatedly said, with tears in his voice, that at last he found a place where he could get to himself. But I suspect his most important work went on outside sessions, out of view.

He linked getting to himself with my honesty. He felt lucky beyond belief to be with someone he experienced as honest. In thinking about this now, I feel honored by Smith. I suppose the cynical me can note how lucky I was to be honored by the sublime Dr. Smith: how flattering to be the only honest man in the world! I needn't tell you I'm no more lily white than you are, my reader. But I do feel honored to have played a role in helping someone die better than he otherwise might have. I suspect many therapists have discovered that our work blossoms at the moment of death. Smith needed me as his *true self counterpart*, and through this projective identification or bit of mirroring, he located a missing area of self.

If Smith was able to use something in me to find a new face, a more honest face, thank God. I feel grateful to reciprocate his gratitude. I can picture Smith staring inward with the worn semi-leer he never fully shook off. As he stares, he sees the face of true self stare back at him, with a smile and wink, gazing through him to the horizon, the eternal opening.

In the last months I saw him, Smith spoke of a peace he never knew before. He was still alive and tortured and striving. But he also felt a deep peace, a reconciliation. He made the link that needed to be made. His insides found features he could recognize in a way that could not be wasted or twisted by words. I suspect what he found could not be communicated, except to say that he found it.

In the last dream Smith reported, a black cat vanished through a basement window into the darkness below. We didn't interpret the dream. The session flew by. I looked forward to seeing Smith again after the weekend. He died walking to the subway after a full day's work.

Where the Force Goes

Where did the force go? Guilty me says it worked in my failure to interpret Smith's final dream. Perhaps if I said the right thing, Smith would have lived a little longer. The dream obviously was about death. Did the cat get my tongue?

Fie on you, guilty me! Thank God Smith's cat went through the basement, rather than Smith going through the roof.

Yet I believe the force was active to the end and beyond the end. As Bion suggests, it goes on acting after it destroys time, space, and existence. The force does not stop in the face of reconciliation, peace, or atonement. If anything, these barriers increase its fervor. Goethe made things too easy for Faust by depicting the inevitable last-minute salvation. New beginnings need new sets of problems. Goethe was right to end with an image of working the earth, the work that never ends.

The force and salvation stay mixed up to the end. Smith died happy but was never free from misery. As he got closer to death, his ability to live paradoxically increased. He became less able to tilt paradox to one side or the other. To close paradox meant to close his heart. He had a lifetime of practice in closing his heart. Smith's bit of opening and peace opposed a lifetime of bad habits.

At the moment of death, new battlegrounds open. New possibilities mean new conflicts, new tensions, new twists. We do not go from conflict to a conflict-free world. Growth in enlightenment is better than that. The force is not wished away by death.

One can invent interpretations of Smith's death, especially the timing of it. Let us say straight away that it might all be physical: his biological clock ran out. But it is difficult not to entertain more possibilities. Most of Smith's life, the force was happy with Smith's false self, his character, the sets of bad habits we call personality. There was enough life and true self in Smith's false self for the force to feed on (in time, it fed on dead aspects of true-false self, too).

The force plays both ends against the middle and plans for the future. While it focused on Smith's personality, it also made inroads on his body. By the time Smith got around to using a true self counterpart to free sparks of true self, the whole psychosomatic system was ready to collapse. There was not enough viable psyche-soma left to support the true self engagement he reached. The house of cards collapsed around the place where the fire that never goes out might have been.

One can imagine the force feeding on the fire as a new world opens. Smith, and his counterparts, don shapes called choices or habits to try to do a better job. They do not merely start over from the same place. Their wink and twinkle and smile seem a bit wiser, a little more open and caring. They feel good to be on the move.

References

Balint, M. 1968. *The Basic Fault*. London: Tavistock.

Bion, W. R. 1965. *Transformations*. New York: Jason Aronson, 1983.

———. 1970. *Attention and Interpretation*. New York: Jason Aronson, 1983.

Bollas, C. 1989. *Forces of Destiny: Psychoanalysis and Human Idiom*. London: Free Association Books.

Eigen, M. 1984. On demonized aspects of the self. In *Evil: Self and Culture*, M. C. Nelson and M. Eigen, eds. New York: Human Sciences Press.

———. 1986. *The Psychotic Core*. New York: Jason Aronson.

———. 1991. *Coming Through the Whirlwind*. Wilmette, Ill.: Chiron Publications.

Fairbairn, W. R. D. 1954. *An Object-Relations Theory of the Personality*. New York: Basic Books.

Khan, M. Masud R. 1979. *Alienation in Perversions*. New York: International Universities Press.

Klein, M. 1946. Notes on some schizoid mechanisms. In *Developments in Psycho-Analysis*, M. Klein, P. Heimann, S. Isaacs, and J. Riviere, eds. London: Hogarth Press, 1952.

Rodman, F. R. 1987. *The Spontaneous Gesture: Selected Letters of D. W. Winnicott*. Cambridge, Mass.: Harvard University Press.

Weil, E. 1958. The origin and vicissitudes of the self-image. *Psychoanalysis* 6:3–19.

The Still Point of the Turning World

Jeanine Auger Roose

At the still point of the turning world. Neither flesh nor fleshless;
Neither from nor towards; at the still point, there the dance is,
But neither arrest nor movement. And do not call it fixity,
Where past and future are gathered. Neither movement from nor towards,
Neither ascent nor decline. Except for the point, the still point,
There would be no dance, and there is only the dance.

T. S. Eliot, "Burnt Norton"

These words of T. S. Eliot describe in poetic form the creative point of the psyche born of God, where chaos and order coexist in potential and actual form. It is an image of the union of all opposites, where the dance of life begins and ends. The experience of the "still point" may be one of madness or centeredness, depending upon the meaningfulness the ego is able to bring to the experience of this point. "Mad" parts are unintegrated, chaotic parts of the psyche that operate autonomously and unrelated to the conscious attitude. We need our mad parts in order to experience our sane parts. They are gifts of the psyche, representing the cutting edge of new contents that have not yet become accessible to consciousness; at the same time, they are a curse of the psyche, carrying embarrassment, humiliation, humanness, imperfection. Like it or not, these mad parts will emerge and create their

---

Jeanine Auger Roose, Ph.D., is a psychologist in private practice in the Los Angeles area. A graduate of the C. G. Jung Institute of Los Angeles and former president, she is interested in development of theory of analytical process.

mischief. The best we can do is acknowledge their potentiality and develop an attitude of acceptance of their reality and the necessity to address them directly within ourselves, not through our work with others. This paper is intended to explore the experience of the "mad" part of the "sane" analyst as an important element of the analytical process.

I'll begin with a confession of a closely held secret. Beneath a persona of professional competence, ability, success, and all those other qualities that communicate an aura of sanity lies a deep "madness" which I am constantly surprised is not seen, since it feels as if it is my most obvious wound. The madness is this—namely, if I work long enough and remain focused on the tasks at hand, someday my life will be ordered and meaningful. I will feel whole, complete, and be at rest at the still point of the turning world. I have known intellectually that this belief is pure nonsense, madness, which drives me incessantly and robs me of ever feeling good and at peace with myself. Enough is never enough. And what is it I feel whenever I momentarily reach that long-awaited goal, where I cannot see anything that needs to be completed? No letter to be written, no phone call to be returned, no decision to be made? I feel lost, panicked, anything but what I imagine I will feel, which is peace, meaning, creativity. In fact, I drop into the very center of the chaos that lies in my being, which I have tried, like Sisyphus rolling the stone up the mountain, to organize and order by doing. Finally I have experienced and realized the futility of this life-long attitude and the necessity for a fundamental change, which requires making friends, rather than doing battle, with chaos.

The central theme of this material is concerned with the relationship of chaos, meaning, and the ability of the analyst to tolerate chaos without succumbing to the madness and disorderliness that often accompanies such feelings. Chaos is not only an inevitable component of life, but it is always present in actual or potential form. In fact, life is chaotic, unpredictable, and always changing. Chaos as disorder is different from feelings of anxiety that are a response to chaos. As children, we learn routines and various strategies to cope with external chaos. These routines create a feeling of predictability and order in life. In essence, the routines provide an external ego while the child develops an internalized ego that provides the possibility of choice. But the archetypal bases of order and meaning are different, although complementary to each other. I propose that an emphasis on doing may lead to an internal sense of orderliness, but not necessarily meaningfulness. Ultimately, it is only through a direct encounter with one's own chaos of being that authentic, genuine, grounded, and meaningful action in life can occur.

Many of the individuals I see in my practice not surprisingly suffer from this same madness. It is the grandiosity of narcissism which Alice Miller describes in *Prisoners of Childhood* (1981). It is the hidden pain of many successful people. A 38-year-old man described it in these words:

> You know, I've just realized that the way I've convinced myself that I am good is through my behavior. If I'm doing it well then I am good. But if you ask me what I feel, I refer then to my character and that feels bad, empty, chaotic. It feels as if someone once reached inside my body and eviscerated me, like a chicken. All of my vital parts, my vitality has been pulled out by some unknown hand and it is only by doing and accomplishing that I can demonstrate my goodness to another so that they can validate my existence.

A common feature of life for these individuals is an alternation between internal states of feeling nothingness, avoiding the void, and swirling chaotic energy, the psyche *in potentia*. The current literature contains numerous descriptions of this state of being. The "sane" person has learned to contain or form a boundary around these feelings so that they do not intrude into everyday life. As long as these boundaries remain in place and are unchallenged, the individual can function effectively in life. But life becomes an exercise of quiet desperation, meaningless ordering of chores, objects, time, and space, devoid of connection with the deeper meaning and creativity. As Jung wrote:

> . . . the anima and life itself are meaningless in so far as they offer no interpretation. Yet they have a nature that can be interpreted, for in all chaos there is a cosmos, in all disorder a secret order. . . . It takes man's discriminating understanding . . . to understand this. Only when all props and crutches are broken, and no cover from the rear offers even the slightest hope of security, does it become possible for us to experience an archetype that up till then had lain hidden behind the meaningful nonsense played out by the anima. This is the *archetype of meaning*, just as the anima is the *archetype of life itself.* (1954, par. 66)

Both of the conditions of feeling the chaos, or nothingness, can be contained by successful *doing* as described earlier, and for all intents and purposes, no one ever knows the deep core of unformed being that resides within. *Doing* may take the form of rituals, compulsions, empathic understanding of the needs, wants, and feelings of others, as well as the entire range of ordinary behaviors that are socially approved. All of these can be used as subtle strategies for knowing what to do and avoiding the possibility that another's gaze will penetrate the benevolent cover that hides a core experience of confusion and emptiness. *Doing* also provides the illusion of creating meaningfulness and order in the face of chaos. If the person knows what to do that will be pleasing and suitable to the other, then it is evidence that they have successfully deciphered the meaning of the other's messages. Their success in early infancy of having to learn to create their own meaning in the face of an essentially meaningless environment continues to operate into adult life. But it is built on a foundation of nontrust that there is order contained within the chaos and that it is not necessary to impose the order from outside.

Patients who have developed the ability to be empathic may have great difficulty not doing or responding to conscious or even unconscious needs of the analyst. They become the "good" patients who bring in their typed dreams each week with lengthy personal and archetypal amplifications, perhaps an active imagination or two or three, a few drawings, and whatever else the analyst expects of a good Jungian analysand. The analysis becomes a repetition of well-learned patterns in which the analyst/parent's feeling of gratification at having such a good, interesting patient reinforces the dis-ease of doing and creates a greater and deeper gap between the conscious order and unconscious chaos. Eventually something will happen—the analysis will become stifled and devoid of energy because all of the energy falls into the unconscious, or a negative transference will develop which removes them from the loving regard of being the good patient, or the chaos will emerge into the process bringing with it the seeds of new life in the form of a whirling turbulent force that can destroy old structures and ways of being.

After five years of analysis in which the analyst had praised the unceasing products of work one analysand poured forth, the analysis itself had ground to a halt. It became a boring repetition of images, dreams, and an overall sense of futility was present. It had become a meaningless exercise, a re-creation of the early infant–parent relationship in which meaningfulness was equated with parental approval. Then a change occurred—a new analysis began, this time with an analyst who did not reinforce *doing* but rather *being*. Shortly afterwards, the analysand dreamed the following:

Dream: *I am with both of my analysts. They are having a case conference about my condition. My new analyst writes my diagnosis on the blackboard—chronic undifferentiated schizophrenia. I feel both shocked and relieved.*

The diagnosis of the psyche spoke to the tremendous gap between conscious and unconscious attitudes, the long-standing state of undifferentiated split in the psyche. The relief experienced in the dream is a result of feeling seen by the new analyst and that the possibility of healing is contained within the framework of the analysis.

The word *chaos* is defined as follows:

1. Any condition or place of total disorder or confusion.
2. The disordered state of unformed matter and infinite space, supposed by some religious cosmological views to have existed prior to the ordered universe.
3. A vast abyss or chasm (obsolete) (*American Heritage Dictionary*)

The word itself is a Latin derivative from the Greek *khaos*, meaning empty space. Other words that are etymologically related include *chasm* and *gas*. The man quoted earlier described his attraction to women as "I see a certain look in their eyes, it is as if they are gases looking for a way to be contained, and I immediately jump to the challenge. Of course, once they feel containment, then they react to me and get angry and leave." He does not yet realize that the state of the inner feminine is also "gaseous" and chaotic and that until there is more earth and ground within, he will continue to be attracted to these amorphous women seeking definition through others.

Chaos is the primordial state of being, before birth. It is without form, amorphous and fluid. A common feature of creation myths is that in the beginning there was darkness or chaos and out of this passive condition arose an animating principle which begins the active ordering of the chaotic state. The animating principle may be either masculine or feminine. The Judeo-Christian myth of creation begins:

> In the beginning God created the heavens and the earth. Now the earth was a formless void, there was darkness over the deep, and God's spirit hovered over the water. God said, Let there be light and there was light. (Jerusalem Bible, Genesis 1:1–3)

The animating principle of this myth is the Word, logos, which begins the process of ordering the cosmos.

The Pelasgian creation myth begins:

> In the beginning, Eurynome, the Goddess of All Things, rose naked from Chaos, but found nothing substantial for her feet to rest upon, and therefore divided the sea from the sky, dancing lonely upon its waves. She danced towards the south, and the wind set in motion behind her seemed something new and apart with which to begin a work of creation. (Graves 1955, p. 27)

Again, the Orphic creation myth begins:

> Black-winged night, a goddess of whom even Zeus stands in awe, was courted
> by the Wind and laid a silver egg in the womb of Darkness; and Eros . . . was
> hatched from this egg and set the Universe in motion. (Ibid., p. 30)

In these two myths, it is the wind, the turbulence, that is the vehicle for
creation and order of the disordered elements that comprise the chaotic
state. Creation cannot occur in a passive inert state of nothingness. The
idea that the chaos can be ordered via thought before the creative act
occurs leads to a paralysis of process and stagnation.

Contrast these mythic descriptions of the creation of the world
with the description of the creation of a snowflake.

> As a growing snowflake falls to earth, typically floating in the wind for an
> hour or more, the choices made by the branching tips at any instant depend
> sensitively on such things as the temperature, the humidity, and the presence
> of impurities in the atmosphere. The six tips of a single snowflake, spreading
> within a millimeter space, feel the same temperatures, and because the laws of
> growth are purely deterministic, they maintain a near-perfect symmetry. But
> the nature of turbulent air is such that any pair of snowflakes will experience
> very different paths. The final flake records the history of all the changing
> weather conditions it has experienced and the combinations may well be
> infinite. (Bleick 1987, p. 311)

It is the effect of turbulence, the force of converging and diverging
currents of energy that conditions the development of the individual
snowflake, the world, and the psyche. And this turbulence, or spirit, is
the animating principle of chaos.

In alchemy, the active animating spirit was conceived as Mercurius,
"the spirit of water," the "spirit of the stone," a principle of nature.
Mercurius is the primeval chaos itself as well as the boundary of vessel
that contains and gives form to the chaos. In the Pelasgian myth, the
north wind stirred up by Eurynome's dance is caught hold of, and the
serpent Ophion appears.

> Next she assumed the form of a dove, brooding on the waves and, in due
> process of time, laid the Universal Egg. At her bidding, Ophion coiled seven
> times about this egg, until it hatched and split in two. Out tumbled all things
> that exist. (Graves 1955, p. 30)

Ophion is the uroboric serpent that forms a boundary to contain the
chaos as symbolized by the egg and create the necessary incubus for
birth.

A chaotic condition is in need of form. The combination of the
dissolution of the ego together with the experience of the disorder of
the chaos can lead to a feeling of loss of soul, a loss of identity, and

possible psychosis. Jung spoke of the appearance of mandalas as a "compensatory principle of order" to the chaos. In the Visions seminar, he speaks of the wall, or drawing a magic circle, as necessary stratagems for protecting the state of chaos while also containing it. He said:

> One is absolutely lost in the turmoil if one has not an attitude, a certain way of facing the chaotic things that happen. For an attitude, the word *spirit* can be used. One takes action and chooses one's criteria in a certain spirit, and that spirit is an attitude that can be formulated as a principle or a philosophic formula. (Jung 1976, pp. 394–395)

In this same context, he describes the image of an amphora with a flame arising out of it. On one side of the vessel is shown a lion, while a snake climbs up on the other side; both lion and snake, symbols of chaos, are trying to get into the amphora. He comments:

> . . . an amphora is a vessel of a definite form, and a chaotic condition is like a shapeless liquid; the liquid contained in the amphora might therefore symbolize man's desire for definite orientation, it might mean the specific attitude with which man reacts against chaos. (Ibid., p. 395)

During an encounter with primordial chaos, boundaries are essential for the protection and integrity of the psyche. The usual boundaries of the psyche most directly connected to the ego, disintegrate together with conscious attitude. Dream images of vessels such as clay pots, cooking utensils, or caves appear as potential containers for the chaos. Analysis itself becomes a vessel within which the chaos can undergo transformation.

The Structure and Function of Boundaries

Hermes, the trickster god of the Greeks, was the marker of boundaries along roads and between cities. As a newborn, Hermes stole the cattle that belonged to Apollo, even after he had been warned that he would suffer serious consequences. Nevertheless, he did not want to accept limits upon his impulsiveness. But when his trick was discovered, Zeus forced him not only to respect the limits of boundaries, but in turnabout is fair play, also gave him the responsibility for establishing boundaries. The herm, or stone heap with a phallus, represented the god performing his boundary-setting function.

Where there is a boundary, there is both an ending or departure from the known, as well as a beginning, an entry into the foreign, alien, unknown territory of the unconscious. Ancient maps pictured known lands as contained by the uroborus, the boundary between known order and unknown chaos. Monick associates boundary marking with possession and ownership and defines it as a masculine function (1987, p. 78). I believe there are two kinds of boundaries, one of which has the purpose of differentiation and marking of space and time, while the second has the primary purpose of containing and holding. The first is what Monick describes as masculine boundary setting, whereas the second can be symbolized by the uroborus or uterus and which I consider to be a feminine boundary. The uterine wall is able to contract and expand according to the nature of the inner contents, just as the uroborus, either by shedding skin or by swallowing less of the tail, can also adjust to the volume contained within the center. Since Hermes is hermaphroditic, it does not seem contradictory to assume that there would be two distinct but related forms of boundaries contained in the psyche.

The functions of boundaries are to contain, limit, separate, and differentiate the one from all others. They are essential for the establishment of an I–thou relationship. Under normal conditions, we are usually unaware of the presence of boundaries both within as well as at the periphery of the psyche. When the environment contains the possibility of real or imagined threat, either in the form of an intrusion into private space or the possibility of engulfment, then do we become consciously aware of the presence or absence of boundaries.

Many individuals have problems with the establishment of healthy, flexible boundaries. For some, the difficulty represents the attitude that boundaries are rigid, firmly upheld limits, much like brick walls that protect and isolate the hidden contents; for others, the feeling of being different is too threatening, humiliating, or shameful; while for others, attempts to create boundaries have been met with consistent intrusion by significant others, such as narcissistically wounded parents and intimates. Eigen, in *The Psychotic Core*, examines the various theoretical orientations to boundary development, including Federn, Mahler, Balint, Winnicott, and Kohut (1986, pp. 139–68). Tustin describes the nature of the boundary of the autistic child as being of one of two forms: (1) encapsulated, rigid boundaries that create a shield to protect sensitive surfaces from potentially hostile, dangerous, not-me experiences; and (2) confusional/entangled boundaries in which the child is inextricably fused together with the substance of the parent in order to not be separate (1986, pp. 19–27). These two extreme forms can characterize the range of neurotic boundaries developed by many individuals who are not clinically autistic but who nevertheless have elements of a hard shell or undifferentiated fusion with others in situations of perceived threat. When working with patients in analysis, these boundaries may be most evident as forms of resistance, and when they appear it is important to note the way in which they operate to "protect" the integrity of the psyche from the threat of chaos and disintegration.

The setting of boundaries is an organic process. The image I use most often to describe the healthy structure and function of a boundary is that of the cell membrane. The membrane creates a boundary between the internal and external environment, permitting the internal integrity of the cell to be maintained in spite of varying external conditions. There are a variety of mechanisms built into the function of the cell which permit adjustments for increased or decreased exchange with the environment in order to ensure survival. The ability to be semipermeable creates an image of flexibility, in contrast to fixity. When two membranes touch, their reactions have been imaginatively described as undergoing movements such as bending, engulfing, fusing, pinching off, and migrating. These imaginal descriptions of the boundaries of physical cells seem to apply to the movements of the boundaries of the psyche as well. Migration, in the form of geographical distance or emotional withdrawal, is a way of establishing a boundary when closeness is too great a threat to the maintenance of inner integrity. One last characteristic of the physical cell seems of note, namely, that a prominent feature of the cell is extremely high electrical resistance.

My picture of the membrane as a boundary is that it is performing a dance involving constant, subtle shifts in movement which open and close the cell, thereby enhancing or decreasing its receptivity to outside influences. Boundaries become unhealthy when this ability to "dance" is lost, and the boundary becomes rigidly open, or closed, or the resistance becomes so high that nothing can enter from the outside. The following dream of a 45-year-old woman therapist who is struggling to develop healthy boundaries to replace boundaries that were essentially confusional in nature describes the process.

Dream: *I am in a schoolyard. There is a funny, tricksterlike man who reminds me of Pan in the yard. He shows a man how to dance through the chain-link fence that surrounds the schoolyard. I watch in amazement as they dance through the wire. I can see a slight twinge of pain at the encounter with the wire. Although I am fascinated and he offers to teach me the same skill, I am not ready to try it myself. I stay outside of the schoolyard and perform a romantic ballet dance. I feel alone and long for connection.*

The image of a new form of boundary, one which is porous yet firm, is presented to the dreamer. The ego is not yet confident that the pain involved in the process of transgression of the boundary can be tolerated, but the future possibility is shown in the dream.

As long as the established psychic order continues to maintain an acceptable degree of equilibrium between self and other, as well as ego-Self, meaning exists. But often life, inner or outer, shatters the container and demands the formation of a new vessel. With the experience of shattering, the old structures of the personality dissolve into their original fragments and swirl in the turbulent motion of inner chaos or fall into the abyss of nothingness. This moment of ending signals the potential moment of beginning, of creation anew.

Analysis as a Vessel of Chaos

Analysis can offer a process for the *temporary* containment of the experienced chaos while the exploration of the fragmented bits of psychic material proceeds. One aspect of the vessel is the *temenos*, a Greek word used to define a sacred precinct within which the presence of a god could be felt (Samuels, Shorter, and Plaut 1986, pp. 148–149). As a psychological concept, it describes the bounded, protected area or space in which something, or someone, such as a relationship, complex, archetype, or process is contained and held. The shape of the analytic temenos is a product of the two individual psyches that collaborate to form the vessel. Each one contributes to the creation of the temenos in different ways and to different degrees. The boundary of the analytic temenos must be well defined while also being able to expand and contract to accommodate the energies contained within the process. A highly fixed or rigid vessel may provide the feelings of comfort and holding originally experienced as an infant when wrapped securely in a blanket. Fixed times, frequencies, and location for contact provide a secure container for the process. But it may be equally important to provide flexibility for some individuals who experience fixity as entrapment and suffocation of the spirit.

The analyst also provides his or her psyche as an instrument for the work of analysis. The transference may include an unconscious projection of wisdom, order, and meaning onto the analyst or the analyst's particular theoretical orientation. To the degree that the analyst is consciously or unconsciously identified with the ideas of a theory, or any of the many ways to organize understanding of the psyche, the shape of the analytical vessel is preformed and predetermined. Consequently, the process of creation may be limited by theory. Order is imposed upon the chaos from the outside, rather than allowing for the internal order contained within the chaos to develop into consciousness.

There is a long-standing tradition that the analytic relationship takes place in a closed, contained environment — to use the alchemical metaphor, a hermetically sealed vessel:

> there can be no communication with third parties on the part of the analyst, such as routine kinds of sharing information about patients with colleagues or with the analyst's or patient's family. (McCurdy 1982, p. 64)

The closed vessel creates a safe, containing, holding environment in which the psychic material of the analysand can dissolve into its primordial elements. It is a space in which regression of the ego into the unconscious becomes possible. A state of being, defined by Jung as *archaic identity* (1921, par. 741–742), and which Neumann more directly defined as *uroboric incest* (1954, pp. 16–18) is established. This state represents the collision of the masculine spirit world and feminine chaos with the union of like substance with like, a state of incest. Powerful, unconscious energies are activated inside the sealed vessel by which both analyst and analysand are affected. To quote Jung, from "The Psychology of the Transference":

> The patient by bringing an activated unconscious content to bear upon the doctor, constellates the corresponding unconscious material in him owing to the inductive effect which always emanates from projections in greater or lesser degree. (1946, par. 364)

Because of this powerful incestuous pull, it has been a fundamental position of Jungian psychology that an essential requirement to becoming an analyst is to be engaged with one's own personal process. Personal analysis of the analyst is limited by the reality that we are never fully conscious and are as subject to the disconcerting, unsettling effects of chaos as are our patients. It is our very humanness, our consciousness as well as our darkness, that not only heals and wounds the analysand but also creates our vulnerability to being pulled into a state of archaic identity, unconscious incest, with the analysand. If we lose the ability to sustain an observing ego position while engaging the unconscious material of the patient, we are then at risk of becoming lost in the chaos with no direction.

What is this state of archaic identity? Jung uses the term:

> *identity* to denote a psychological conformity. It is always an unconscious phenomenon since a conscious conformity would necessarily involve a con-

sciousness of two dissimilar things, a separation of subject and object, in which case the identity would already have been abolished. (1921, par. 741)

It is the foundation of *participation mystique*, as well as the phenomena of *projection* and *introjection*. It is an undifferentiated state of being, which corresponds to autistic, primitive, infantile states. The critical elements are that there is a lack of differentiation, i.e., a state of conformity/fusion with the other, and that it is an unconscious phenomenon. It is a state of chaos, the *massa confusa* of alchemy, into which consciousness has been dissolved.

The closed temenos of analysis gives permission for the dissolution of the boundaries of the psyche, e.g., ego defenses, thereby enabling the release of the psychic elements from their hidden, private space. The analyst is thereby enabled to have a direct experience of the analysand's undifferentiated state of being. It is through participation in this state of archaic identity that the subtle body (Schwartz-Salant 1989) is formed, or alternatively, the *mundus imaginalis* (Samuels 1989, pp. 143–174) develops. Through the deep, shared unconscious union, transference/countertransference material is generated and provides the basis of our ability to mirror the other. Reveries, fantasies, images arise out of the shared state of being. It is our ability as analysts to participate in this unconscious experience of uroboric incest and to maintain an observing ego relationship that underlies our effectiveness in the work.

One of the dangers of the closed space is related to the development of psychological conformity, which is the shadow state of conscious individuation. It precludes separation, uniqueness, and difference and maintains a condition of sameness with the other. It can become very warm, cozy, womblike inside the temenos. The longed-for state of incestuous merger with mother/father/analyst is finally gratified; no one else, for the moment, is allowed inside without permission. Safe, secure, and held, all boundaries disappear. Unconscious union has been achieved. As long as the analysand conforms to the analyst, or vice versa, this unity can go on undisturbed. But if the individuation process is to develop, there must be a disturbance, a beginning separation of the elements into opposites with the emergence of an I–thou relationship, otherwise the analysis will become stagnant and interminable.

What is the origin of the disturbance? Under most circumstances, it comes from the "still point," the animating energy of the wind, or the word that begins the active ordering of the chaos. The breaking up

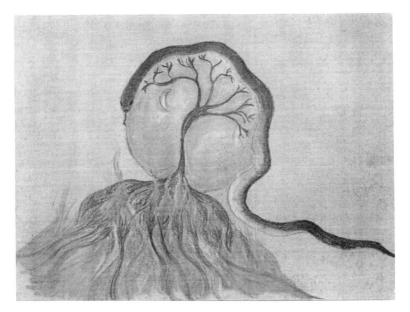

Figure 1.

of the uroboric temenos signals a new birth of consciousness and differentiation. Figure 1 is a spontaneous image drawn by a woman analysand. Our analytical work had begun approximately three years prior to
this drawing. She felt intense anxiety in connection to the image, which
I understood to be the pending breakthrough of the chaos contained by
the snake, now in the process of unwinding. Her drawing reflects the
infusion of fire and passionate feeling from the breast/mountain/earth
into the rarefied, ethereal realm of thought and intuition. Such fire
and emotion are necessary ingredients for the work, for the problem of
chaos is usually at the level of feeling, not thought. The sky is split into
two halves by the tree, a Self symbol rooted in the body of feeling,
which grows from the earth into the previously contained space that,
until the snake unwound, only contained the crescent moon. Clearly a
process of growth and differentiation is beginning. This image was
followed by major life changes. Whereas she had been "stuck" and
unable to initiate change, she now began to have the energy available
for change and action. At the same time, the analytic relationship
changed from one that was predominantly mirroring to a form that

began to demand more human, personal involvement on my part. I could be more present as a separate individual in the analytical work.

What if the disturbance does not develop naturally from the psyche? This may be a point when the possibility of termination or working with a new analyst may be considered. In my paper, "Images of Endings" (Auger 1986), individuals reported that a primary motive for termination was a feeling of being stuck. An analysis of dream images associated with negative termination experiences, as valued by the analysand, revealed three general themes: (1) negative images of the analyst; (2) encounters with a new analyst/guide; and (3) being on a dangerous journey alone through a swamp or body of water. The last group of images underscores the experience of feeling lost in the chaos without the presence of a guiding spirit or attitude.

A second alternative may be to do the very thing that Hilde Kirsch said is not allowed, namely, deliberately break the seal and let fresh air into the vessel. She writes of such an experience in "An Analyst's Dilemma." She had planned to present an active analytic case to a professional seminar without informing the patient. She writes:

> My natural tendency would have been not to present this case to the Clinic, especially as I know the attitude of the Zurich analysts and Institute about not presenting any material of an analytic process which is not yet finished. (Kirsch 1961, p. 171)

Kirsch does not say why she selected this case, but perhaps there is a clue in the following passage:

> I hesitated about presenting this case, because she was rather boring. Very little had actually happened in her analysis, in her dreams, and in her conscious life. Nothing touched her. . . . By now I had great doubt that anything would ever happen to her. (Ibid.)

This description of the work sounds as if they were locked in an eternal incestuous embrace of archaic identity.

The first event that happened was that the patient brought a dream to the next session that spoke of a break in the analytic container. Later, Kirsch had a spontaneous active imagination in which she took a steamroller and:

> going with it through a brick wall, it was as if an ironlike barrier broke down and finally I could get to the other side. . . . I suddenly felt free to go ahead with the case presentation and prepare the material. . . . I certainly did not expect the dramatic development that occurred . . . as a direct consequence of my intervention. In the very next interview, the patient was completely changed. She looked happy and free . . . the hard brick wall that had always surrounded her had disappeared. (Ibid., pp. 172–173)

Kirsch clearly places the wall/boundary/barrier inside the patient. But I think a more likely hypothesis is that the act of breaking down *her* own inner brick wall, namely, the Zurich rule, was what freed the energy of the psyche. There was too much archetypal material floating in the uroborus with no ego present for a personal connection.

A third alternative is to continue in the state of incestuous embrace and pray that eventually the gods will intercede. The following material relates to just such a situation. My focus will be on my participation as analyst in the chaos. But first, a case summary.

Phil is a 51-year-old single male whom I have seen for ten years. He was referred following an arrest for drunk driving. He had been sentenced to attend an educational program for convicted drunk drivers that included five sessions of individual counseling. The counselor recognized that Phil's characterological problems were a major contribution to his alcoholic behavior and felt he would benefit from further counseling.

Phil was adopted at age 6 months by a well-to-do couple living in the Midwest. Two years later, his sister was born. Although he denies any feelings of abandonment, loss, or sibling rivalry, the rage present in his nonverbal behavior is enormous. He is psychotic and helpless; ego consciousness is virtually nonexistent; every hour is an encounter with chaos.

His entire life pattern is a repetition of early childhood: a complete and total lack of motivation to do anything, overt compliance with the wishes of the parent and simultaneous covert rebellion against the wishes of the parent. Because he has been able to develop a likable persona, he has managed to go through life with everyone accepting his helplessness. At the same time, he is able to come up with unique solutions to problems. For example, when he was living in New York City, he could not find a laundromat. However, he remembered that he had an airline credit card, so he bundled up his laundry, flew to Chicago, and went to the laundromat near his former apartment.

Phil's helplessness is total. Because of a trust fund, he has not had to work for a living and was able to purchase a home with money that he inherited. His living environment is a direct reflection of the state of his psyche. The house is filled with old newspapers, magazines, videotapes, records, broken television sets, inoperative stereos, an answering machine that doesn't work because rats chewed the cord, a hole in the roof that rain pours through; the few social contacts that he has retained avoid entering his house because of the overwhelming mess. Over and over, he says, "I need someone to help me clean it up. I am so embarrassed," yet when friend directly offer to help, he refuses because they will not do it on his terms. He asked me to come see his house and the way that he lives, and I finally agreed but stipulated that it was necessary that he do something about the rats because I was uncomfortable with the idea of being in a house with rats. He managed eventually to destroy two of the three rats, but their function as objects of relationship overrode his desire for me to see his living situation.

As far as I can see, his life situation has deteriorated steadily over the ten years he has come to see me. He has no dreams, no imagination, a total lack of empathy. His main focus is on sleep, which occurs during the daytime hours and which he says is the only order in his life. His contact with me, two times a week, is the only other activity that occurs with some predictability in his life and is the only one that requires him to leave his house.

It feels as if I am locked in a death grip. No matter what I do or say, or do not do or do not say, nothing changes. When we are together, I have fantasies of striking matches, sparks, of the need for something to animate or activate the psyche. I referred him for a psychiatric evaluation to determine if there might be some type of medication that would help provide the needed spark. He took Prozac for six months and began to sleep 20 to 22 hours a day, instead of the usual 10 to 12 hours. He demands that he be fed what he wants and in precisely the manner that he wants, at his total control. I am a puppet, and he is the puppeteer. Sitting with him for two hours a week is a humbling experience. I have given up the idea that I am capable of helping bring him to life, to the state of being that he says he wants but which every action on his part sabotages. We are firmly fixed at the "still point."

Yet the madness I revealed at the beginning of this paper continues its seduction. Perhaps if I listen carefully enough, for a long enough time, if I do not give up my belief that ultimately transformation and change will occur, then order and meaning will emerge out of this meaningless process. My omnipotence is not that of God's, I am unable to speak the word and "let there be light," nor can I dance and stir up the wind to give birth to life and eros. Logos and eros are absent from the process.

Recently, Phil did not appear for four consecutive sessions. Periodically, he will miss one or two sessions because of his rage at having to do something in order to come to my office. But this was unusual. The first three he called to give an excuse, the last one being that he had showered, eaten breakfast, and then felt dizzy so he was not going to come. When I did not hear from him the next time, I felt concern.

Although he has been given a clean bill of health, he expresses a large number of unusual or weird body symptoms. Given the fact that he lives alone and that his most recent message included the symptom of being dizzy, I thought there was a possibility that he was at risk and might need help. I had a fantasy of calling 911 and sending the paramedics to his house. I didn't act on the fantasy, because I believed that, in fact, he was not in danger. But as a symbolic statement, I do believe that the situation is an emergency. He is literally in need of resuscitation, of emergency care. When I told him my fantasy, he felt angry with me for two reasons: first, he would have felt such total embarrassment at having strangers break through his door into the chaos in which he lives; and second, if I really cared, I would have come over to his house myself. He is, of course, right. I have moved beyond caring, to the point which he remembers his mother expressing when she would say, "Phil, please don't tell me about your life, I can't stand it anymore." Initially, I reacted with judgment of his mother when I heard this plea; now I understand her feeling more compassionately.

What possible meaning is there in having such a person in my practice? This paper is the creative product of my chaos which I experience with such immediacy two times a week. If it were not for Phil, I could continue to believe that meaning and order are attainable states given sufficient time and attention. Jung spoke of the archetype of meaning; Phil connects me to that aspect of the archetype that is meaningless and chaotic.

In *Memories, Dreams, Reflections*, Jung said:

> The world into which we are born is brutal and cruel, and at the same time of divine beauty. Which element we think outweighs the other, whether meaninglessness or meaning, is a matter of temperament. If meaninglessness were absolutely preponderant, the meaningfulness of life would vanish to an increasing degree with each step in our development. But that is—or seems to me—not the case. Probably, as in all metaphysical questions, both are true: Life is—or has—meaning and meaninglessness. I cherish the anxious hope that meaning will preponderate and win the battle. (Jung 1961, pp. 358–359)

Phil is wholly neither-nor. There is little differentiation between conscious and unconscious. The problem with Phil's analysis has been that he and I have colluded to contain the chaos of his psyche within manageable limits, but in that very choice to contain—he via a passive/helpless/polite persona, and me via an unconscious push to order—we had constantly poured water on the animating principle of his psyche—his deep, sadistic, infantile rage. Phil was involuntarily hospitalized at age 18 by his parents, and he is desperately afraid of this experience being repeated. He himself is afraid of his own rage and potential destructiveness and has split off the collectively determined persona from his internal reality. But the rage emerges in explosive, destructive ways, through antisocial behaviors including alcohol abuse, shoplifting, stealing from friends, failing to pay taxes, excessive withdrawals from his trust fund, destruction of property, rebellious rejection of help including the conscious rejection of analysis and the analyst, refusal to reflect on material between sessions, and failure to come for scheduled appointments. He is a young, unformed infant who unceasingly cries for his mother's breast and when it is offered, he bares his teeth and crushes the nipple relentlessly.

Why do I continue to see Phil? For one reason, because he comes and in coming expresses a degree of hope. There is a therapeutic connection in which, to the degree that he is able, he experiences trust and understanding, discriminated caring and acceptance. He keeps me honest and humble—I've suggested that he see someone else but he refuses to do so. And lastly, he has been abandoned by every single significant person in his life, beginning from birth—that fact alone weighs heavily.

Entering one's own chaos, or the chaos of another, requires a willingness to experience what Tillich writes of as encountering the ontological anxiety of emptiness and meaninglessness—a confrontation with the possibility of there being no-thing, no-being within that provides meaning or ground to one's Self (1952, pp. 46–51). Absence of being, in the sense of authenticity, results in a life determined by collective forces. The genius of Jung gave him the courage to enter the chaos of his being and discover meaning, which he then communicated to others. Ultimately, authentic meaning is grounded in the uniqueness of one's Self as experienced through the ongoing effects of the turbulent dance of life. It is a meaning that embraces both the "mad" and "sane" parts of the psyche and engages life to its fullest. The tragedy of Phil is that he has become one with the turbulence, the turning world, while he yearns for the still point of inner peace and centeredness.

References

Auger, J. 1986. Images of endings. *Journal of Analytical Psychology* 31:45–61.
Eigen, M. 1986. *The Psychotic Core*. Northvale, N.J.: Jason Aronson Inc.
Eliot, T. S. 1943. *Four Quartets*. New York: Harcourt, Brace, Jovanovich.
Gleick, J. 1987. *Chaos: Making a New Science*. New York: Penguin Books.

Graves, R. 1955. *The Greek Myths*, vol. 1. New York: Penguin Books.

Jung, C. G. 1921. *Psychological Types. CW*, vol. 6. Princeton, N.J.: Princeton University Press, 1971.

_____. 1954. Archetypes of the collective unconscious. In *CW* 9i:3–72. Princeton, N.J.: Princeton University Press, 1959.

_____. 1946. The psychology of the transference. In *CW* 16:163–323. Princeton, N.J.: Princeton University Press, 1966.

_____. 1961. *Memories, Dreams, Reflections*. New York: Vintage Books.

_____. 1976. *The Visions Seminars*, vol. 2. Zurich: Spring.

Kirsch, H. 1961. An analyst's dilemma. In *Current Trends in Analytical Psychology*, G. Adler, ed. London: Tavistock Press, pp. 169–175.

McCurdy, A. 1982. Establishing the analytical structure. In *Jungian Analysis*, M. Stein, ed. LaSalle, Ill.: Open Court, pp. 47–67.

Miller, A. 1981. *Prisoners of Childhood*. New York: Basic Books.

Monick, E. 1987. *Phallos: Sacred Image of the Masculine*. Toronto: Inner City Books.

Neumann, E. 1954. *The Origins and History of Consciousness*. Princeton, N.J.: Bollingen Series, Princeton University Press.

Samuels, A., Shorter, B., and Plaut, F. 1986. *A Critical Dictionary of Jungian Analysis*. London: Routledge and Kegan Paul.

_____. 1989. *The Plural Psyche: Personality, Morality and the Father*. London: Routledge.

Schwartz-Salant, N. 1989. *The Borderline Personality: Vision and Healing*. Wilmette, Ill.: Chiron Publications.

Tillich, P. 1952. *The Courage to Be*. New Haven, Conn.: Yale University Press.

Tustin, F. 1986. *Autistic Barriers in Neurotic Patients*. New Haven, Conn.: Yale University Press.

Sectarian and Titanic Madness in Psychotherapy

Rafael Lopez-Pedraza

It was while I was preparing this paper that I began to realize just how much of a challenge the theme of this Chiron conference is for me. The title "Mad Parts of Sane People in Analysis" points to a shadow: as if, in the practice of an analysis that strives for healing and sanity, there is another side which is madness—a mad shadow.

I am going to discuss some aspects of this mad shadow which have been haunting me, aspects that undoubtedly belong to my own psychic wounds. I have always felt that psychotherapy, as I prefer to call it, cannot be talked about in a direct way. In my books, *Hermes and His Children* and *Cultural Anxiety*, I used an indirect approach, and issues such as sanity and madness stayed in a hermetic borderline where they were contained and less polarized. It is for this reason that the theme here is such a challenge for me, because it impels me to discuss directly the madness hidden in so-called sane people.

The title also contains a fundamental pair of opposites—"mad" and "sane." If the most rudimentary aim of psychotherapy is to arrive at

---

Rafael Lopez-Pedraza was born in Cuba and studied at the C. G. Jung Institute in Zürich. He is currently a lecturer in mythology at the Central University of Venezuela, where he also conducts a private practice. Previous books include *Hermes and His Children* and *Cultural Anxiety*.

a livable balance between our madness and our sanity, then this theme offers a thought-provoking field for reflection.

My concern in this paper is sectarianism and titanism, two components of human nature that I propose to discuss in relation to "Mad Parts of Sane People."

My reflections on the psychology of sectarianism owe a great deal to Euripides' classical tragedy *Hippolytus*, which provides an archetypal background. Hippolytus is the paradigmatic model of the virginal, puritanical personality prone to sectarianism. Hippolytus makes his first entry on stage in the company of a group of huntsmen friends, singing a hymn of praise to their patroness, Artemis:

> Follow, and sing!
> Follow the bright Daughter of Heaven!
> Follow our guardian Maid,
>   Artemis!

Dear Mistress, I am your companion, speak with you, hear your voice; only your face I do not see. And may the end of my life's course be as the beginning! (p. 29)

Later, when the tragedy has unfolded, Theseus, Hippolytus's father, in an extraordinary speech which has always puzzled the scholarship on Hippolytus, accuses his son:

So you—you are the man above men who keeps the company of gods! Yours is the chaste life unsmirched with evil! Who believes your bragging? Who charges gods with such ignorance and folly? Not I! So, now flaunt your purity! Play the quack with your fleshless diets! Take Orpheus for your lord and prophet and wallow in frenzied adoration of his wordy vapourings! (pp. 55–56)

These two scenes can be seen as complementary in their portrayal of the virginal, puritanical personality. The first can be seen as an anthropological image of the sectarian. While the second, Euripides' reflection of Orphic sectarianism put into Theseus's mouth, can be seen as an image of the civilized sectarian. Is not the latter evocative of the modern manifestations of this archetypal pattern? Before leaving Hippolytus, we should take into account two ingrained characteristics of his personality: his exclusive loyalty to Artemis, with its resulting rigidity, and his contempt for and brutal rejection of everything that does not pertain to his goddess. "And may the end of my life's course be as the beginning" is the expression of a nature which, archetypally, does not seek any psychic movement.

Martin P. Nilsson, in his discussion of Orphic sectarianism, writes:

> It was the creation of a religious genius, but it took place among a people whose psychology permitted them to react very little to the sense of guilt, and was enveloped in a mythology which could not but be repulsive to that people's clear processes of thought. (1949, p. 217)

The passage from *Hippolytus* gives us a classical archetypal view of sectarianism. Now we have Nilsson's reflection that sectarian guilt, in classical times, was alien to the pagan spirit, a reflection confirmed by Theseus's rejection of his son's Orphism.

To turn to sectarianism at the time of the rise of Christianity, E. R. Dodds writes:

> We have the descriptions of a number of ascetic communities which appear to have sprung up independently in different parts of the eastern Mediterranean shortly before the time of Christ: Essenes in Palestine, Therapeutae round Lake Marreotis, the Egyptian contemplatives described by Chaeremon, and Neo-Pythagoreans in Rome. (1965, pp. 30–31)

There has been a great deal of speculation, though little scholarly evidence, about the Essenes' influence on the life and teachings of Christ and his followers. In an "age of anxiety," these sects flourished, an indication that historical moments of severe psychic upheaval are propitious for the sectarian spirit and way of life to catch and give form to the excess of suffering and anxiety. It is clear that, directly or indirectly, the spirit of sectarianism was flourishing at the beginning of Christianity and, in a variety of ways, has continued to be important throughout history. Today, in another age of anxiety, either within the spirit of Christianity or outside it, the phenomenon of sectarianism has erupted again, catching and containing an excess of suffering.

Now let us take a look at an image of a modern sectarian. I shall call him A. He is a 45-year-old lawyer—tall, asthenic, and gaunt, with a big head and long beard. He had been divorced two or three times and had various children. But the pillar of his life and philosophy was his Indian guru, who he went to see in India whenever he felt his psyche was in a deep crisis or on the verge of breaking down. During the first hours of his psychotherapy, he told me that, while on a visit to Mexico, he became accelerated after seeing too many Mexican images. He was high up in a bell tower when he realized that he was in pretty bad shape and suddenly remembered that a friend had told him about an ashram in Los Angeles. Whereupon he took a plane to Los Angeles and entered the ashram. Immediately, he began to feel calmer and in better shape. It was obvious that the sect, or his transference to the sect, gave him a certain psychic balance. His contact with a sect, the aspect of the archetype his psyche required for its basic balance, activated in him a ritualistic communication and restored his equilibrium.

Apart from his dependence on the sect, his personality contained a strong element of anorexia nervosa. He spent a great deal of time talking about diets. He even had the fantasy of solving the world's food problems with a diet based on the soybean.

It was not difficult to realize that he came to see me because there are no ashrams in Caracas and, at the time, he had no money for going to India to see his guru. My psychotherapeutic attitude was to find a symmetry with what he brought to the psychotherapy. It is fundamental to my conception of psychotherapy to bring a symmetric approach to the patient. It is by being symmetric that communication comes about. Mythologically, I attribute symmetry to the constellation of Hermes and Pan, and it is through this constellation that the psychotherapeutic "dance" becomes possible, as I wrote in *Hermes and His Children* (1989, p. 136). So I treated him as if my consulting room was an ashram, and we engaged in what I took to be a model for conversations in an ashram. By being receptive to his conversations about his Indian guru and encouraging him with my curiosity, he was able to find the necessary balance to embark on what were his real conflicts at that time.

This analytical experience with A shows in a nutshell how quickly the psychology of sectarianism works. Almost immediately it catches and contains a psyche which is on the verge of breaking down. A is for me the sectarian per se. I cannot imagine him being able to live without having a connection to a sect and the amenities it provides, such as meditation, breathing exercises, macrobiotic diets, amulets, etc.

Although A is a typical case of the modern sectarian, the catalog of sectarianism is varied. I had another analysand, a young man who, when he was 26 years old, was hit by a very complex family tragedy. In the middle of the emotional turmoil he was going through at that time, almost unconsciously, he joined a sect, where he remained, suffering a great deal of guilt and inner conflict, until he was 35 years old, at which time he came into psychotherapy with me. He had been so suffocated by the sect that the first part of his analysis was wholly taken up with discussing sectarian psychology. His experience demonstrates again just how rapidly sectarianism can hold a psyche that is under the pressure of extreme suffering.

Here I would like to mention that I was acquainted with a young man who, being unable to bear the adventure of the shadow in Jungian analysis, joined a very rigid sect in order to cope with his psychological conflicts. Another acquaintance, although he never actually joined a sect, knew a great deal about the ideas and way of life of many sects. I have the impression that, in this way, without the literalization of joining an actual sect, he was feeding his psychic need for sectarianism.

Today, the efficiency of the sects in treating addictions is well known. The sectarianism of Alcoholics Anonymous is patently able to hold the madness of addiction to alcohol, where psychiatry and psychotherapy have failed. And we have all met those people who spend their lives in an endless peregrination from sect to sect, desperately trying to find the perfect container for their sectarian psyches.

Jung spoke about religious and esoteric sects — how they are a net in which to catch the madness of people who, otherwise, would have to be interned in mental institutions. His famous remark, "Thank God I am Jung and not a Jungian!" was perhaps a reference to modern psychology's sects. I am doubtful, however, whether Jung was fully aware of the implications of sectarianism, and of his own suffering at its hands. In spite of Jung's telling remark, I think we can agree that modern psychology has not discussed sufficiently the psychology of sectarianism and the sectarian shadow in the different schools of modern psychology.

The study of man's psyche and modern psychotherapy were born under the sign of sectarianism, a historical fact that has made for a strong influence lasting to our own days. As soon as modern psychotherapy began — a discipline that was meant to open up a new adventure into the psyche — it was taken over by sectarianism.

The first wave of psychoanalysts were bound in obedience to the founder of the school of Vienna, whose studies became the laws of the sect which the adept must not transgress. Classical psychoanalysis functions as an orthodoxy. The sanity of the analyst is not in question. He has been analyzed himself, has learned a technique, and belongs to the Society. Classical Freudian analysis is the perfect model for sectarianism in analysis.

Then came Jung's break with Freud. I am going to limit my view of this rupture to its sectarian aspect: to see it as an outcome of sectarianism and as an image from which to have an insight into the early appearance of sectarianism in modern psychology. We have to appreciate that, at the time of the break, psychology was still profoundly influenced by the natural sciences. So, after the break, emotions were hidden by long theoretical discussions to explain two different scientific views.

In *Hermes and His Children*, I reflected the break as the expression of a polar split between Freud's adherence to power and Jung's hermetic nature (1989, p. 33ff). But now we can look at Freud's insistence on his "authority" as the jealous power of the leader of a sect. Sectarianism is built on obedience to the founder and the rules of the sect. To leave the sect makes for an unavoidable feeling of guilt: Jung the dissident, to use the label ideologists give to make the dissenting person feel guilty. The times were not yet propitious for Jung to say to Freud, "Listen, we are two totally different people. Our natures are simply different." This sort of attitude would have made all the difference between a sectarian view of the situation and an individual view.

Sectarianism is archetypal. Apparently the archetypal energy at the roots of sectarianism generates the enthusiasm for the aims and way of life of a sect, as can be mirrored in the anthropological image of Hippolytus singing in praise of Artemis with his huntsmen friends. The main activity of a sect is to sing in praise of either a god or goddess, a guru or leader of the sect, or even of the rules underlying the sectarian way of life. However, it was Euripides' genius that showed the other side of the coin: how fanaticism came into play and brutally repressed all that ecstasy and fulfillment. Hippolytus repressed everything to do with other gods, especially the carnal Aphrodite, and the result of this was tragedy—the death of Phaedra and of Hippolytus himself. Greek tragedy gives us the proper background for reflecting the destructive consequences of extreme and fanatical sectarianism: the rejection of everything that does not pertain to the ideas of the sect, as has been all too evident throughout Western history.

I have always held strongly to the individuality of the psychotherapist, disregarding the school he or she belongs to: the practice of psychotherapy as the meeting of two unique psychic entities. It is an attitude that is in opposition to that of sectarianism. So, here, things become slightly more complicated. Sectarianism is archetypal and so invites a state of unconscious identification, and such states can be stubborn and hard to shift.

One of the ways in which sectarianism can creep into our practices is through the use of Jungian semantics. Terms such as *anima, animus, shadow, persona, Self*, etc., are so taken for granted that they become passwords of the Jungian sect and block the analyst's recognition of the analysand's real psychological troubles. Unconsciously, a subtle pressure is brought to bear on the analysand to become an adherent of the Jungian sect or one of its branches. But it is not only the analyst's sectarianism that we have to be aware of; we all know of the many people who go into Jungian analysis already well versed in the theories and semantics of their school and predisposed to experience their analysis and psychological studies as a sectarian way of life. And I am aware that my own standpoint of the individuality of the analyst, although it may not be contaminated by actual outer sects and trends, may still contain this archetypal, virginal, puritanical component of our nature.

In my book of essays, *Cultural Anxiety*, I introduced titanism as a subject for psychological discussion. In this paper, my aim is to see how titanism appears in analysis in both analyst and analysand. About the Titans, Kerényi wrote:

> The stories of the Titans are about gods who belong to such a distant past that we know them only from tales of a particular kind, and only as exercising a particular function. The name of Titan seems originally to have been the supreme title of celestial gods, but gods of very long ago, still savage and subject to no laws. (1961, p. 20)

> Hesiod told us that Father Ouranos had given them the name "Titans" as a term of abuse and as a pun, as if the word were derived from *titainein*, "to overreach oneself," and from *tisis*, "punishment." (Ibid., p. 207)

The etymology of the word *Titan* shows what the Greeks thought about titanism: excess and punishment for that excess. In historical times there was no cult of the titan, no representation and therefore no communication. Thus the primordial roots of psychotherapy and transference—ritual and communication—cannot function in relation to titanism. This would be the psychological premise for detecting the presence of the titanic component in analysis.

We all have a measure of titanism in our nature, although controlled to some extent by the many other rituals which give form to our lives.

The psychology of titanism is difficult to discern because of its overwhelming historical reality in the world today. We live in the face of more and more titanic excess in all areas of life. So the reality of living in a titanically driven world, whether for survival or destruction, affects us all and, psychologically, where it affects us most is in the function of reality (Janet's *fonction du réel*). We are lucky if we have the energy to keep track of all the changes required of us, without being overwhelmed by or identified with the excess which can blunt or destroy our feeling function, the reservoir of our individual values.

The titanic personality is a rare bird in psychotherapy, so when one does appear, it is tremendously welcome. I would like to introduce an analysand I have who could be said to be an exemplar of a titan in psychotherapy.

Let us call him B. He is 46 years old and a very successful entrepreneur. B was sent to me by his physician who, while unable to find any physical complaint or illness, was worried by B's excessive way of life. B could be termed physically healthy and sane, although his appearance belies this: he is invariably pale and has a demented, possessed look.

Most of his time and energy go into his various businesses, which seem to be managed in a somewhat chaotic way. He once showed me his appointment book, in which three different lunches had been scheduled for the same time. His social life consists of frequent parties at which business conversations have priority. Recently, his son, who is a baseball fan, invited him to a lunch to meet some baseball players. Afterwards he commented to me that it was the first lunch at which he had talked to people without mentioning business or money. And yet, I do not get the feeling that he is really interested in money like other entrepreneurs, who have a sense of what the traditional values of wealth could mean. Neither does his striving to make money seem to be backed by any fantasy of power, such as those entrepreneurs who measure their power by the number of shares they hold in a company. His businesses seem to be simply the expressions of his titanic madness. One feels his psychic poverty in spite of all his success in life, a success the collective would consider to be the fruits of a sane personality.

In Jungian analysis, it is usual to assess the patient's psychological situation through a notion of space and time. It is this sense of space and time that enables the analyst to see when a complex is constellated and to place that complex historically. Now, in the titanic personality, there is a very peculiar relation to the dimensions of space and time. In the case of B, daily outer activities rule his existence and become almost a state of possession: a frenetic acceleration, an excessive velocity without limits. The three lunches scheduled for the same time are evidence of a disturbance in relation to time and space. This sort of disturbance becomes even more evident when the titan travels abroad. Just to follow the itinerary from city to city and country to country produces vertigo: all notions of space and time are transgressed. This velocity invades all areas of B's life: he is always on the go, and the notion of taking a break and relaxing—fishing, playing golf, going to a spa, etc.—is completely alien to him. All this frenetic activity is accompanied by an extraordinary rhetoric, making the diagnosis of titanism inevitable. I am using the term *rhetoric* here not only as it applies to speech, but also in the broader context of the accelerated, titanic way of life.

It is in this wider conception of the titanic rhetoric that I find the ground where I can put myself in some sort of therapeutic symmetry with B. Symmetry happens in the many conversations about his businesses and business relationships. And it is here, in this symmetric familiarity, that there is the possibility of constellating psychological slowness. From the beginning of his therapy, B has had many dreams that express his need for incubation. Through a symmetric approach, I am able to adjust myself to these dreams and to encourage him, with all my imagination, to seek the rest and incubation he so obviously needs.

But we must not delude ourselves: the titanic component is also to be found in the studies of psychology and the practice of psychotherapy. There is the titanic conception of futurism, for example. I am acquainted with a psychotherapist who is convinced that, in the future, there is going to be a "true" psychotherapy. His main interest is in the most recent contributions to the field, and he is certain that each one is more advanced than its predecessor, that is to say, nearer to his futuristic vision of the perfect, healing psychotherapy.

Then there are analysts who are in a state of titanic possession, which a friend of mine graciously coined as "furor curandis": the conviction that all psychic states of whatever gravity can be treated and cured. If in psychotherapy we cannot distance ourselves from this sort of titanic excess, then what is really mad and ill seems to be sane and healthy. It is, of course, easy to understand that, however good our psychological antennae may be, the demands and pressures of outer titanic reality have an impact on us. When titanic outer reality imperceptibly encroaches on the analytical consulting room, and the analyst's intention becomes the promotion of a better and saner therapy, then psychotherapeutic reality is turned into madness.

We cannot learn how to practice psychotherapy when we are taken over by the velocity of the titanic drive. Psychotherapy is an inner activity, and it takes many years of practice to assimilate any depth. We can presume that a great deal of the process of learning about psychotherapy is, like any other learning process, through imitation or mimesis. This is probably a consideration of great importance for the theme of madness in psychotherapy. We have all seen the mimetic use of psychotherapeutic schemes, concepts, and theories, a titanic mimetism which is not adjusted to any psychotherapeutic reality.

Now let us try to explore a gigantic shadow in psychotherapy, a shadow I see as being composed of three components: titanism, psychopathy, and power; components that, phenomenologically and semantically, tend to be confused. Titanism has a mythological legacy, as we saw from Kerényi's description of the titans; and owing to its predominance in the world today, of the three it is the component that most distorts our sense of reality.

Psychopathy is a deficiency, or a "flaw," in human nature. We are not complete, we have psychopathic lacunae, or "black holes," where no imagination is possible. Nothing comes out of the lacunae, except possibly psychopathic mimetism.

Of the three shadow components we are differentiating, I would say that power has the most direct effect on human relations. Jung saw it as the exclusive opposite of eros. When power manifests, there is no possibility of eros. In an interview, Jung said also that when power appears, the sense and meaning of what is being dealt with is distorted and becomes something else. Adolf Guggenbühl-Craig (1971) has seen the appearance of power as a sign that the archetype is not functioning. In order to write about the very difficult issue of power, both Jung and Guggenbühl-Craig have had to fall back on a Christian concept—the *privatio boni*, the absence of good, in this case, the absence of eros.

We do not talk much about the madness of power; however, I see it as the expression of a madness, but one which cannot be affiliated with the psychotic madness of the psychiatric textbooks or with the mental illness it is possible to treat.

As analysts, we have to be alert to a manifestation of power in our analytic practice, such as being overwhelmed by the analysand's power drive and responding with the same drive. In a situation like this, the analysand's health becomes secondary, for the analyst's own health is at risk in the practice of a repetitive, guilt-making, power-ridden psychotherapy.

Now let us take another look at sectarianism and titanism to see what they can tell us about power. Sectarianism is archetypal, as we have seen, and the activity and behavior of a sect can become fanatical. Probably, when we see the excessive zeal of fanaticism taking over the archetypal configuration of the sect, we can begin to suspect a power drive is at work, destroying the forms that contain the sect.

In the May 6, 1991, issue of *Time* magazine, the cover article, entitled "The Thriving Cult of Greed and Power," is a report on a sect which calls itself the Church of Scientology, a sect about which I knew nothing before reading the article. It so happened that I was immersed in writing the last part of this paper when I read *Time's* investigation of Scientology and immediately saw its pertinence to the subjects of sectarianism and titanism. *Time's* description of Scientology is shocking. The conception of the cult can only be likened to the sort of delirious fantasy elaborated by a mental institution's most peculiar and paranoid patient. But how the sect operates is another cup of tea. Its purported aim is to "clear" people of their unhappiness, but, in reality, it is a devilish machine of extortion.

In *Prometheus Bound*, Aeschylus, with poetic irony, presents the titan Prometheus as a god, but a god whom Zeus has had bound to a rock in chains as a punishment. Prometheus personifies the component of titanism we all have, the titanism of which it is so difficult for us to be aware. The binding of Prometheus suggests that the titanic nature, with its rhetoric, can only be reflected upon and understood when it is immobilized. Throughout the play, Prometheus displays a boastful rhetoric in which he defies Zeus and attributes to himself all the benefits given to man for his survival. At the same time, it is a rhetoric in which one senses an undercurrent of power. In claiming to be man's benefactor, as with most benefactors, there is an autonomous drive for power at work. There seems to be a strong link between titanism and an autonomous power drive.

Perhaps here would be the place to distinguish between power and authority. Prometheus's claim to be the benefactor of humankind disguises his drive for power. Archetypally, each god and goddess has the authority pertaining to his or her godhead. But I think we could say that Zeus would be the archetype par excellence exemplifying authority in contradistinction to power. And it is precisely this authority that Prometheus is bent upon dethroning. Aeschylus gives us a picture of what power is: a desperate longing to destroy authority.

To finish this paper, let me quote a few lines from the close of Aeschylus's play, which are relevant to our theme. Before the final destruction, Zeus's messenger, Hermes, after listening to Prometheus's rhetoric (statements such as: "I am one whom he [Zeus] cannot kill") and trying to bring Prometheus to reason without success, comments to the chorus in words that can be taken as a diagnosis of Prometheus's psychological condition:

> Thoughts and words like these
> Are what one may hear from lunatics.
> This prayer of his shows all the features of frenzy;
> And I see no sign of improvement. (1961, p. 51)

Hermes makes his clear diagnosis in the first two lines. In the third line, he includes the titanic component of frenzy. But the last line of his speech is the most pertinent to the theme of this conference—"And I see no sign of improvement." In a situation such as this, Hermes is an authority, since we know that, traditionally, he was one of Aesculapius's teachers. He sees there is nothing more to be done.

Prometheus is a tragic figure with whom the audience is prone to identify. Like the chorus, we empathize with the suffering of the chained Titan. But Prometheus's suffering is repetitive. It is a repetitive, titanic suffering pointing to a part in human nature which does not change. Titanic suffering is very different from that of Psyche, for her suffering brought her to psychic awareness and love.

I feel that a great deal of madness is present in psychotherapy when the analyst, unaware that there is a part in human nature which does not change, insists on trying to improve, or heal, what cannot be improved or healed. Often the family, or society, or even the analysand demands a change in that part of the analysand's nature which does not change; likewise, there are analysts who put all their effort into trying to change that same unchangeable part. I consider this unconscious projection upon healing most likely to constellate titanic power in analysis: the insistence on redeeming what is irredeemable, or, to put it in the traditional language of Western culture, on saving the soul at all costs, including burning at the stake.

References

Aeschylus. 1961. *Prometheus Bound*. Philip Vellacott, trans. Harmondsworth, Middlesex, England: Penguin.

Dodds, E. R. 1965. *Pagan and Christian in an Age of Anxiety*. Cambridge: Cambridge University Press.

Euripides. 1953. *Hippolytus*. Philip Vellacott, trans. Harmondsworth, Middlesex, England: Penguin.

Guggenbühl-Craig, A. 1971. *Power in the Helping Professions*. Zürich: Spring Publications.

Kerényi, C. 1961. *The Gods of the Greeks*. London: Thames and Hudson.
Lopez-Pedraza. R. 1989. *Hermes and His Children*. Einsiedeln: Daimon Verlag.
_____. 1990. *Cultural Anxiety*. Einsiedeln: Daimon Verlag.
Nilsson, M. P. 1949. *A History of Greek Religion*. Oxford: Clarendon Press.

Naming the Nameless

Mara Sidoli

In his recent paper, "Jung's Infancy and Childhood and Its Influences upon the Development of Analytical Psychology," Brian Feldman wrote:

> While Jung's early experiences had mainly an ecstatic emotional quality, this emotional tone may have been a defence against a particular painful affect. The source of this pain was apparently the significant problems with Jung's family. When Jung was three years old, his mother was hospitalized for what appears to have been a severe depression. She was away from the child for several months. During that time, he was taken care of by a maid.
>
> At that time, Jung developed a severe skin rash which he later on connected with the separation of his parents and his mother's separation. It is probable that the skin eczema was related to the sense of psychic catastrophe which Jung experienced subsequent to his separation from his mother. It was as if he were unable to contain tortuous emotions within himself and they burst out in a somatic form. (1992, p. 262)

Then Feldman quotes Jung:

> I was deeply troubled by my mother being away. From then on I always felt mistrustful when the word *love* was spoken. The feeling I associated with woman was for a long time that of innate unreliability.

Mara Sidoli is a Jungian child and adult therapist in private practice, on the clinical faculty of the University of New Mexico in child psychiatry, and president of the Jung Institute in Santa Fe. She is the author of *The Unfolding Self* and the forthcoming *Incest, Incest Fantasies, and Self-Destructiveness in Adolescence*, which she is coediting.

Feldman goes on:

> I think that the passage quoted above may help us in understanding the
> origins of Jung's difficulties in his emotional relationship with women: his
> need to make sense of the nonsense of his mother's breakdown and long
> absence, and the pain that it caused him, for which it seems that he received
> no emotional help at the time, and by which he was 'deeply troubled.' He
> seems to have experienced his mother's hospitalization as a betrayal which led
> him to be "always mistrustful when the word *love* was spoken."

The question is: Could baby Jung have been helped in making
sense of his mother's illness? Could he have been made to understand
that her leaving him was not a betrayal? Did anyone tell him that his
mother loved him, that she was miserable because she had to go away,
and that she was aware of the pain and panic her departure caused
him? What part did this early abandonment contribute to his difficulties and his own breakdown in later life and could it have been allevi-
ated by someone talking to him about it? It is difficult to say a poste-
riori, but early dramatic experiences of the sort he underwent are a
significant factor in the activation of early splitting defense
mechanisms.[1]

I will write about two patients, Andrew and Linda, who, in my
view, did not receive sufficient contingent maternal support to make
sense of their experiences as a small child, and thus parts of their
personalities remained in a state of confusion, panic, and despair.

As Jung said, ". . . meaninglessness, and the lack of meaning in
life is a soul-sickness whose full extent and full import our age has not
as yet begun to comprehend" (Jung 1934, par. 815).

Andrew

Autistic — Do Not Speak

. . . My words are lost shouts in a dead prison,
torn assemblages of thoughts in a mute body,
Or dust in the air that breathed then.
My words are stones sweeping the beach,
The pebbles thrown carelessly by innocent children,
Sinking.
Swept away
By the tide.
All worn and inadequate communications.

Broken mirror: Darkened windows.
Empty shells on the shore—You can hear the sea.
But I who is words, untrained passion and solitude,
I am unaccessible, unexpressable, floating unwritable thoughts,
They are my movements and my body . . .

Andrew was an articulate and sophisticated 17-year-old. He came from an educated, intellectual family. His mother was a doctor of medicine and his father a university professor. Everyone in his family was highly intelligent and articulate, and knowledge meant everything to them. Andrew had one older brother.

When Andrew first came to me, after having rejected another therapist, he was suicidal and greatly distressed, but for many sessions he kept up a steady stream of cool, sophisticated, and matter-of-fact conversation about education, literature, and theater, which were his hobbies. He was bright, entertaining, and witty. He spoke at great speed without ever losing the flow of the conversation, as if he were afraid of letting go of the ball for fear of losing it to the other team or not scoring. His words flowed endlessly, as if intent at leaving no gaps, no empty spaces during which he might catch a glimpse of his own distress and loneliness. He seemed to be keeping himself together by stringing interminable chains of words, while his body sat stiffly in his chair, like a wooden puppet.[2]

Andrew's use of language seemed to have a defensive quality to it right from the start. I believe that his lively conversation had several aims: one was to make himself interesting and to communicate his ideas; another, less conscious one was aiming at concealing his feelings of vulnerability and inferiority.

Could his need to develop mastery of language from an early stage have emanated from his need to be understood by his intellectual and professional mother? Did baby Andrew use words to reach his mother in order to involve her with him? He also used sounds as autistic objects in order to make himself feel alive. Sometimes he used words as empty shells, merely for decoration; at other times, he used words as "stuffers," to fill up empty gaps of time and space between us, especially when he felt in danger of falling into a frightening hole where his shouts and screams would get lost. The early internalized mother was a noncontaining, nonsoothing "dead prison" in his mind.

In my countertransference, it became clear to me that I was not expected to absorb, contain, or hear anything he was telling me. I felt as if I were not there, as if he were talking to himself in a sort of masturbatory way, puffing himself up, listening with obvious pleasure to the sound of his own voice and showing off his verbal acrobatics. Through my feeling of being shut off by him, I could be in touch with his sense of hopeless loneliness.

Looked at from an oedipal position, his stiff body posture suggested that the boy was in a permanent state of erection with emotions/meaning attached to it, as if in his adolescent mind he was still unable to make sense of these bodily feelings and emotions for which the early mother had not provided a containing name.

Right from the start I was struck by the split between the animation in his voice, the liveliness of his speech, and the lifeless rigidity of his limbs. At the beginning, he hardly ever moved in his chair. He often sounded like a headmaster reporting—with poise and superior arrogance—on the problems he was having with one of his students. The "headmaster" was a personification of a stereotyped rigidity which he was trying to emulate and was criticizing at the same time. The stiff persona, which he mistakenly identified with "adult behavior," was also often attacked by him in these reports, but only when he allowed his adolescent self to come through.

It seemed as if the male role model offered him by both the headmaster and his own father, the university professor, had a rigid quality to which his own personality could not adapt, in spite of his sincere attempts to fit in with their demands. He was a playful, lively child who had been mercilessly repressed and undermined. This repression was partly a collective repression, due to the British educational system in which he had been raised. But it became clear to me that his personality would never fit into that particular mold without great loss of creativity and joy of life.

On the other hand, his connection with his mother as a small child had also lacked closeness and warmth, due in part to her own personality and to the fact that for long periods of time he had been left with a variety of caretakers while his mother was at work.

He did have a good, warm connection with a grandmother, as well as—later on—with his father, who used to spend a lot of time at home writing. Yet even then he was not allowed to go talk to him or to disturb him with his boisterous, enthusiastic stories, because the father needed quiet for his work.

All of this became slowly clearer to me through his talking and my observation of him, session after session. While he was swamping me with his endless speech, I had to hold on to my thoughts. Often I found myself thinking "after all, there is nothing wrong with this young man, he is okay." Then, however, I would remember that this same young man had tried to commit suicide. Obviously, I was getting caught up in his splitting. He wore the conversational persona as a mask and wanted to make me and everyone else believe that, indeed, he was all right.

Unfortunately for him, the same defensive system was operative in the very culture in which he lived. Thus, he had to go a long way before his despair could come to the fore and manifest itself in the suicidal behavior. The feelings which he described in the poem — "I who is words, untrained passions and solitude, I am unaccessible, unexpressable, floating unwritable thoughts, they are my movements and my body"—slowly became available to be worked on in the analytic sessions, and in my work with him I concentrated on the analysis of the material with a particular focus on the preoedipal aspects. Thanks to our work together, he was finally able to feel the depth of the split within which he was operating, as well as make sense of and give a name to his deepest emotions. These emotions were all the more disturbing because he never knew that they were there. They were "movements in my body," nonspecific discharge of restless discomfort.

These nonexpressible states of discomfort are, in my view, related to untransformed early infantile experiences which have not been made sense of, primarily by the mother, in the dyadic relationship. The empathic tuning in with the infant on the part of the mother and her maternal care has two aspects: one is the physical attending to the baby's body, the other is the attending to the baby's emotional needs. The empathic tuning in on the part of the mother usually alleviates the infant's sense of impotence by promptly meeting his needs in a manner that the infant can experience as "magical" or "miraculous."

This may sound all too complex, but most mothers are naturally able to perform this function and, on the whole, these complex interactions take place in an average way within most mother–baby dyads. But a variety of factors may hamper the smooth development of this mutuality: illnesses, deaths in the family, and premature separations of mother and baby (like his mother returning to work too soon, as in the case of my young patient).

In my view, which was confirmed by my countertransference, Andrew's mother was only partially able to decode the nonverbal communications of her baby. Often in the sessions I felt like a baby, completely nonexistent; he was constantly talking above my head. I felt undermined, uninteresting, as if he were not paying attention to my words. I felt frustrated and ignored, just as baby Andrew must have felt, unable to communicate his feelings to his mother.

The feelings that he was evoking in me were those that he had kept inside himself, raw, unprocessed, and loaded with violent emotions of which he was unaware. In his analysis, he kept projecting these feelings onto a girlfriend, his headmaster, and me. These primitive, unintegrated parts of himself reemerged due to the developmental crisis of adolescence (the deintegration of adolescence, according to Fordham) and had started exerting pressure on his ego and needed to be integrated.

At first, Andrew had tried to deal with the problem by using the splitting mechanisms by which he had operated in those areas since infancy, but with the energy liberated by the upsurge of adolescence, his earlier mechanisms could no longer protect him from the painful, distressing bad feelings which had been locked up in the unconscious meandering of his bodily experience. The last lines of his poem describe this state of affairs very well: "I am unaccessible, unexpressable, floating unwritable thoughts. They are my movements and my body."

However, the poem I have quoted here was written by him in the third year of his therapy. Only then was he able to express the state he had been in and give it a name. At the beginning of the therapy, he appeared to want to impress me with his manners, his intellectual and verbal abilities, and most of all he wanted me to treat him as an equal. In this way he would be just as attractive as any oedipal rival, like his brother, his father, or any of my other male patients. In reality, he felt he was the least "interesting one," the baby with the small penis in whom either his mother or I could not possibly be interested. On the other hand, as a defense, he had adopted the "stuck on" grown-up behavior which had made him very unpopular with his peer group, as he "acted grown up and arrogant towards them." In relation to me, I think that he had wanted to distract me, to make me find him interesting, an equal, a man with a "big penis" like his father, thus using oedipal fantasies to cover up earlier infantile ones in relation to the preoedipal mother and her early abandonment. His experience had been of having to hide and strap in the part of himself which felt "inaccessible and unexpressable."

As I mentioned, I could only vaguely intuit this state of affairs when he first came to see me, but many images of bleak, derelict, empty houses appeared in his dreams at the onset of his therapy. He also complained of feeling bored and lonely and of spending a great deal of time locked up in his room alone, listening to loud rock music. He had managed to split off his worst feelings, projecting them onto a girlfriend who, as he told me, had tried to kill herself, and he had become very concerned on her behalf. We spent many sessions in which he described his girlfriend's extreme feelings of emptiness, despair, and loneliness. He depicted her household as cold and bleak and said that nobody loved *her* at home. The more he progressed in the description of the girlfriend's emotional state, the more I would become aware of him projecting his vulnerable, infantile, distressed part onto her. But it took a long time for him to be able to see what he was doing. I also felt that in the transference he needed to experience me as a mother/ girlfriend who could engage with him emotionally, understand him, and contain him without falling apart.

However, the transference of his sexual fantasies into me, mother/ girlfriend, aroused great anxieties and excited bodily feelings in him, as whenever he talked about his girlfriend in the session, he could no longer maintain his rigid body posture. He would become agitated and begin to move his body with jerky restlessness on the chair. He interspersed the descriptions of the girlfriend with reports of his activity in school and his teacher's complaints about his "noisy restlessness," which disturbed the lessons.

An interesting coincidence was that another patient of mine accidentally broke the chair in which Andrew used to sit. It came unglued, and I had to send it out for repair. Andrew immediately noticed the disappearance of "his" chair but did not verbalize it. Instead, he exhibited a distressed state which he could not attribute to anything that had happened to him. He looked anxious, became completely stiff, appeared agitated and unable to sit comfortably; I pointed this out to him, but he was unable to make sense of what was going on. This behavior carried on for a couple of sessions during which he regressed considerably, looking insecure and depressed, and complaining that he did not know what was going on with him. At the same time, he seemed to scan me with the greatest attention, to control my every movement, as if he were expecting some dangerous reaction from me.

Actually, I thought that the disappearance of "his" chair (and the unconscious meaning that it had for the infantile part of him) might have been the factor that had caused his regression. At an oedipal level, his reaction might have also been caused by the fantasy that a male rival had been inside me in his place.

However I chose to interpret that, it seemed to me that what he was feeling was related to his unconscious anxiety about having destroyed my chair/me. He feared being a bad, destructive boy, like as an infant he had feared having destroyed his mother's lap, which caused his mother to go away, and he had felt abandoned and desperate. And now he was afraid that he had damaged me, too, and that I would abandon him also. At first, he verbally rejected my interpretation; but his body immediately began to loosen up. He sat more comfortably, leaning back into the chair, and all his body tension disappeared. He resumed his lively conversation and seemed to enjoy the remaining part of the session.

It was only some sessions later that he was able to tell me that I was right. He *had* worried about the chair. He was afraid that I would get angry, and that my husband (the oedipal rival) would get angry with him, too, and that we might ask his parents to pay for the damage. The same thing used to happen at school, where his parents were constantly called in to hear complaints about his lack of discipline.

The episode of the broken chair and his regression and panic reaction in the transference made it possible for me to have a reverie and fantasy about how he had felt as a small child, apparently blaming himself for his mother leaving him. It also brought into the open his fear of his father's anger and punishment for his misbehavior.

In the countertransference I felt his preoedipal fear and panic at the thought of having damaged the mother's/analyst's lap/chair, mixed with his castration anxieties about the revenge of the oedipal father (my husband). By interpreting these feelings to him and naming them, I helped him to make sense of nameless emotions, which had remained raw and unprocessed because his mother had been unable to tune in and give a name to the negative feelings that he had experienced as a baby when she had returned prematurely to work.

Thanks to the transformation produced by the naming of the emotional state of the past, which gave relief in the present, the experience became digestible, and Andrew slowly began to make sense of his early history as distinct from the present.

A few months before his therapy ended, after his final exams, Andrew decided to go on a trip to the Far East, which we understood as being his initiation quest. The trip went well, and I would like to quote here a passage from a letter he wrote to me from India: "No one hustles or feels the need to rush about—this is partly to do with the heat . . . however, I have felt a new kind of stillness and see the beauty of waiting with the right mind of being calm and serene. This only leaves the problem of how to balance this with my more boisterous side. I have not found it particularly easy to be away from home. I feel that I have done only so that I can be welcomed back and thereby judge their love for me. However, on the other hand, there have been times again when I have felt stronger than I have ever done before — being almost alone and winning — I am able to cope with this, though I am occupied more with new ideas from the very Indians I have talked to on trains."

In this letter Andrew was reassuring me that he was okay in spite of the hardships that he was having to face in his journey. He also acknowledged to himself that he missed me and his family, and that being away from the home he had complained about was a mixed blessing. He realized he loved his parents and me and regretted being away, although he had to for his own needs. He was telling me that moving away and separating both from me and his parents was not just the "good riddance" experience which he had fantasized about, but by being away he could miss the good aspects of home and therapy and enjoy the idea of coming back.

This meant to me that he was now really ready to leave therapy as he had reached the ability to leave experiencing grief, and he could tell me about it.

Before going on to the next case, let me say this: the ability to communicate with words is a specifically human quality which is slowly developed in the first two years of life. To be able to use words and language is the first step in the process of symbolization by which a person or a thing is called and designated as distinct from another person or thing. It is the only way by which one's personal experience can be made accessible and transmitted to other human beings, by the use of a shared symbolic code.

Before words begin to exist as a means to express oneself, sounds and actions have to be used to make oneself understood. From birth, babies address themselves to their mothers and/or parents expecting to be understood and have their needs met, and they are endowed with a variety of facial expressions and gestures to communicate their emotions and interest. On their part, the parents have the difficult task of helping to translate into language these nonverbal communications. The function of helping the baby put into words his experiences and give them a name is a very complex one which demands empathic tuning in on the part of the adult. By helping the baby to find words for experiences and emotions as yet unnamed by him, the mother facilitates the baby's dialogue with the world, as the baby can share more effectively his feelings, needs, and thoughts.

Under normal circumstances, a baby is able to make sense of his experiences and to receive support from his mother in states of anxiety, pain, distress, or whenever he feels overwhelmed by frustration and fear. However, there are great differences in babies and their inborn capacities as well as in mothers and their mothering abilities and their sensitivity to the baby's communications and needs.

There are circumstances in which the flow of communication and emotional exchange between mother and baby are disturbed for a variety of reasons, such as the baby's fragility, or the mother's insensitivity, or external events such as traumas, premature separations, illnesses, or death. In these cases, those areas of emotional experiences often remain unnamed because the baby has no words for them.[3]

In order for the mother to experience this "reverie," she has to be able to make space inside herself for the baby's emotional evacuations. She needs to contain them, sort them out, and return them to him enriched with meaning. However, many factors may hamper this process: if the mother is depressed, ill, or her mind is taken up with preoccupations and worries of all sorts originating from her family or working life, for instance, she will not be able to dedicate to her infant the amount of reverie that he needs. This in turn will lead to difficulties in tuning into her baby's nonverbal communications.

One might say that, for instance, in the case of Jung, when the maternal "reverie" failed to perform the transformation for the baby, the beta elements remained raw and primitive and manifested themselves as disturbing, unintegrated "crazy parts" in an otherwise functioning psyche. These (psychotic) beta elements are often not verbalizable and manifest themselves in somatic form as well as in uncontainable affects and grandiose fantasies. In Jungian terms, we may say that these primitive elements — which he called "psychoid" — have remained in an asymbolic, unnamed form.

I, on the other hand, believe that the fundamental function of the analyst, when working with regressed patients, consists of helping them to name and make sense of these primitive unnamed elements (Bion's beta elements), which block and disturb their emotional development. In so doing, the analyst can be helped greatly by countertransference reactions and emotions.

In my own work, I am very attentive to nonverbal bodily communications on the part of the patient as well as to my own countertransference reaction to those nonverbal communications, in order to try to penetrate the misty area of preverbal interaction and relatedness. To do this, one needs to focus one's attention on every minute detail of the session. Not only does one need to listen to all the verbal communications and silences, one needs also to perceive all the changes taking place in the patient's body, such as vitality levels, breathing patterns, tension levels, and voice changes, and one needs to let oneself be tuned in with them in one's own body in order to relate them to the emotional states of the patient of which he himself is not conscious. From the subsequent reflection and evaluation of *all* the data thus collected, the analyst will hopefully be able to construct a useful interpretation in due time. My second case history will illustrate further.

Linda

Linda was in her early fifties when she was first referred to me. She was an attractive woman who looked a great deal younger than her age. She was slim, moved gracefully, and had an unconventional way of dressing — somewhat like a hippie — which often made her look like a teenager. There was an air both of great determination as well as fragility about her which reflected her inner state. At times, she coupled the look of the femme fatale to that of an innocent baby which was both disarming and alarming, given her age. At times she reminded me more of a delicate flower susceptible to withering at a mere touch than of a woman of flesh and blood.

At the time she came to me, she had been divorced for some years. She had two adolescent children who had given her a number of problems, but overall she had cared for them very well. She was involved with a boyfriend much younger than herself with whom she had a sadomasochistic relationship. She was fairly successful in her profession as a student counselor. She had trained as a visual artist but suffered from "painter's block" and had recently applied to train as a psychotherapist.

She often complained about her difficulties with "boundaries," getting overinvolved with her students — letting them stay in her house for months on end without paying. She would try to please them in every possible way, overidentifying with them and feeling — and often actually being — used by them rather than acting as their counselor. She was also aware of problems in personal relationships where she would tend to lose her own self into the other.

Her childhood had been full of the most distressing and dramatic events. Her parents were aristocrats and could be considered dreamers, in love with each other, with beauty, and with art. Her father was a sculptor. Her mother, who had married at seventeen, had always led a sheltered life and was incapable of coping with reality. Their romantic love affair turned into a disastrous marriage, as the sculptor was drafted into the Navy and left to fight in World War II after just a few years of marriage.

After struggling to survive with two babies (my patient being the eldest, and her brother nine months younger) and trying to get help from various men friends, the mother decided to send the children away to a children's home and get herself a job. By that time, my patient was barely four and her brother three years old. Shortly after the parents divorced, the father was assigned custody of the children while the mother, feeling lost and helpless, fled back to her own country from which she planned to regain custody of the children with the help of her own powerful family. In the meantime, however, the political climate had changed in her country, and she found herself trapped behind the Iron Curtain, unable to contact her children for many years. After her parents' divorce, my patient and her brother, by now six and five years old, were sent to live with a paternal uncle who lived in the country.

Thus, by six years of age, my patient had had to cope with separating from 1) her father, at one year of age when he went to war; and 2) her mother, at age three when she was sent to the children's home; and at the age of six, having lost her mother for good, and having to adapt to life with a couple of practically unknown relatives. Moreover, until the age of three she had only spoken her mother's language — her father found this "cute."

Linda told me: "My father and mother both idealized me, calling me their beautiful little angel, adored me, and seemed not to have the slightest idea of my real needs. At three I was sent away from home and from mother. I found myself totally in a foreign land, as I did not speak English. I could not express myself, and the only familiar person there was my little brother."

The two of them clung together for dear life. It seems that, in the chaos of her life — both internal and external — she held herself together by identifying with the maternal role in relation to her younger brother, thus projecting the baby onto him and taking care of him and her own "inner baby" in projection. The connection with her father, to whom she was very attached, was inconsistent. She was completely deprived of news about her mother, whom everybody believed dead. Still, she managed to keep a certain steadiness.

Her brother committed suicide in his late twenties. At that time, her world collapsed. She had a serious depression which necessitated hospitalization and had been struggling with ups and downs ever since. The episode of the hospitalization surfaced well into the course of the therapy. In the first sessions, she conveyed to me a feeling of great distress and extreme loneliness while appearing polite and competent. She was cautious and seemed not to care at the same time.

At the time she came to me, I knew that I would be leaving the country three years later, and from the first interview I told the patient that I did not feel it would be a good idea to start working with me, as it would have repeated the situation of her early childhood with her mother. Yet I found her workable and did not want to reject her. She seemed disappointed but went away without protesting. She left it at that for a while, but some time later called me back and told me that, in spite of what I had told her, she had had a good feeling during the interview, and she knew that she needed to work with me, even within the time limit that I had given her.

I was hesitant at first, because I thought that my departure might precipitate a crisis related to her early losses or that the notion of it might prevent attachment. But after talking the problem over with a colleague in supervision, I realized I had felt some positive personal qualities in her and had been moved by her story. I decided to take her on. But I kept in mind the limitations, imposed by the circumstances, which constellated right away on the theme of loss.

We started working three times a week, and she developed an idealized transference which served to protect me from an equally negative one that she projected onto the aunt who had brought her up. Thus, right away, the two aspects of the mother archetype became split and projected with extreme passion: the good one onto me (otherwise she would have been unable to attend analysis) and the bad witch onto her paternal aunt and a series of women "outside there." I was aware that having mentioned at the very start my future leaving was what had intensified the constellation of that type of transference. She needed to idealize me, to deny and displace any negative feelings against me, the mother/analyst who once again was going to abandon her baby self.

Yet she had wanted to work with me, she had chosen me. From the idealized mother I would also often become the good father, and I felt that she needed to recreate a couple of good parents and leave the bad one out of the room and tell me about them "outside there." Anything else would have been too dangerous.

Linda worked with extreme determination and persevered with great intensity, which reminded me of an infant who vigorously latches onto the breast. Each session was intense and left me feeling depleted and often confused; such were the needy, chaotic emotions that she put inside me in projective identification.

It took a long time and was quite difficult to decrease the idealization and to make her understand that she referred to the aunt's cruelty, particularly at times of breaks or when she became anxious following some interpretation that she experienced as particularly persecutory.

To induce her to stay with her feelings of loss about her mother and the suicide of her brother without hating me for bringing it up and then letting her go after the session was hard and painful. Fortunately she was endowed with great resiliency and defensive denial, which helped her to deal with the extreme amount of pain and despair slowly, in order not to break down. To name so many losses would have been too much for anyone, let alone making any sense of them. On the positive side, which I never failed to emphasize, she *had* been a good mother for her children despite innumerable difficult circumstances, and she was successful in her work. She told me that she wished the analysis would enable her to establish a better relationship with her mother and to manage to forgive her. After the death of her brother, her own marriage had gone to pieces, her father died a squalid death, and she lost her aunt and uncle. In the meantime, however, her mother had reappeared, and she and Linda had reestablished some flimsy contact.

I would now like to report here one dream that Linda had a year and a half after starting analysis, which points to the split between the happy-looking, graceful girl and her underlying despair. The dream occurred during a Christmas break, when we were not seeing each other, and she felt the need to post it to me, as it scared her. During breaks, she was always terrified that I would disappear or die, and also that she had caused it to happen, as she had always imagined—as a child—that she must have been so bad as to drive her mother away. Therefore, breaks were the times when her inner turmoil and infantile feelings were most likely to surface and, for this reason, we had agreed that she would keep in touch by mail, and I would acknowledge receiving her letters, so she would know for a fact that I was alive.

Dream: *I was on the top floor of my father's large house in London. I had to leave. I put on my pink satin shoes, tied the ribbons around my ankles and walked beautifully through the house — round and round and down — walking like a ballet dancer all the way. I kept passing artists whom I either knew or had known — I had to walk through their spaces, which was taken for granted. They all watched me walking and thought that this was fascinating and beautiful. I knew this. But there seemed to be another whole, lonely person being carried around on these feet—waiting for someone to come and take care of her whole body—but no one realized that because she walked with such confidence. And so they let her walk by.*

I went into the street, which was desolate (it was the area where my father used to live). The sun was shining. I walked. I think I was walking back home. There was no one in the streets. Then I was somewhere near my home, walking across the common, when I heard four explosions. I looked at the sky. I thought something horrible has happened and was about to happen to us. I called out for my boy friend—we must run for cover—he was some distance from me. But it was too late. It was impossible to hide. I saw the whole building—it was a synagogue—flying slowly and menacingly through the air on its side, like a rocket. It was very very frightening. I didn't know whether it was going to explode or whether it was going to crash on me.

Next thing I knew it was gone. I was still walking wearing my ballet shoes through town. I had a black felt tip with a wide tip and every bit of writing on the building (which curiously seemed all to be producing cakes and pastries of some kind) I was underlining—I knew this to be vandalizing. Then I thought how difficult it would be to remove the ink and how I was spoiling the face of the buildings which made me feel sick anyway—all those bakeries . . . how disgusting that everyone eats so much cake.

Starting with the next session, we worked on this dream for many weeks. It was an important dream, and Linda had felt so, but she could not make sense of it herself. She had the dream during my absence and wrote it to me. I interpreted that the dream seemed to contain all the elements of loss and abandonment which she had experienced earlier in her life, and that it had been triggered by the break and my abandoning her over the Christmas holidays. The house of her father where she used to spend her holidays was empty. The streets were deserted. She felt that nobody realized (meaning that I did not realize during the session) how bad she had felt as she walked with her ballerina shoes with such apparent confidence. The ballerina dancing away is a representation of her persona and her manic defenses, aiming at denying the pain and experiencing some comfort by an activity she liked, being able to function as she had to when she was a child and nobody had been there for her.

In the second part of the dream, after the patient becomes aware that the streets are deserted, that there is no one there for her and that she has been abandoned, the explosions take place. There are four explosions, and as we remember, she was four years old at the time of the first abandonment and great danger. These explosions were also actual memories of the bombing of London which had terrified her as a child and could not be interpreted exclusively as psychotic material.

In the dream she fears that she is going to be crushed by a synagogue flying through the air. She had often thought that I was Jewish and asked me about it repeatedly. Her rage is completely split off and comes back at her with the image of a potentially deadly blow that will crush her, because as a child she had witnessed several bombings of London. The explosions are realistic enough, as well as her fear of being blown up.

However, in the dream she uses the image of this event which is out of her control, as she is not yet able to connect the explosions to her deepest feelings of frustrated need and rage reactivated by the abandonment in the transference. Thus, she put on her brave-ballet shoes-manic defense and denial and she carries on dancing. However, some of the anger and destructive revenge is acted out by messing up the buildings with the black felt tip and by complaining that the sweet food makes her sick (the breast has turned bad).

This dream took up many sessions, as her long dreams usually did. We had to struggle with her splitting which prevented her from owning up to her own feelings, and her denial of admitting any destructive, revengeful feelings against me for fear of acting them out and actually hurting me.

A few months later, when she allowed herself to feel angry at another one of my holidays, she told me (although she was frightened doing so) that during my absence she had come by my house and thrown big stones at my garage door, and that now she knew that the dream had spoken correctly about her wish to mess up/vandalize the bad mother/analyst-breast whom Linda had felt rejected by.

Discussion

The excerpts from the two analyses which I have presented here are different in many ways, but they are similar in the fact that both patients were not able — before entering analysis — to name and make sense of some deep, troubling distress that disturbed their daily lives. Both of them experienced abandonment on the part of their mother in early childhood, although in Andrew's case there seemed to be a more definite noncontingency on the part of the mother in relation to his infant self.

In Linda's case, there had been a prolonged breast-feeding stage and close connection with the mother for at least the first three years of her life which, compounded with her natural resources, seemed to have been just enough to support her under normal circumstances. She experienced a complete abandonment at four years of age, at which time I feel she was better equipped than Andrew had been to identify with the good mother role. He seemed to have a more brittle ego than Linda's.[4]

However, I believe that another variable is the actual age of the child when abandonment is experienced, in order to understand how things went wrong. Also, the position in the family is important in understanding how feelings of self-esteem or lack of them may complicate the situation in relation to narcissistic injury. For instance, Andrew felt that he was the youngest, least significant member of his family, whereas Linda was the valued, idealized little angel of her parents' dreams. Although this image is highly charged by archetypal projection, it still contains more positive projected fantasies on the part of the parents with which Linda could identify when she dreamed of the beautiful ballerina dancing in her silk pink shoes. I believe that the fact that she was the first child and had been able to take care of her younger brother had rewarded her ego as a child and helped her to value herself through an identification with the hero archetype. One might hypothesize that her brother, who seems to have had a more fragile nature and, on top of that, was younger at the time he was sent away, could not manage life and committed suicide in late adolescence.

My analyst training, combined with my experience of real infants but mainly my countertransference reactions, helped me to tune in with these patients' early needs and anxieties which had remained split off and unknown to their adult egos. Thus I was able to perform the reverie that their mothers had not; that is to say, experience within myself their chaotic, primitive emotions, recognize them in myself, and name them to my patients.

Notes

1. Bion states that psychotic states are defensive protections against "thinking the unthinkable" and experiencing psychic pain, and they result from the nontransformation of beta elements into alpha functions. Beta elements may be correlated to the very first

deintegrates of the primal self (Fordham) and are as much psychic as physical. According to Bion, alpha elements are those that contribute to the development of the alpha function which presides over the symbolic area of thoughts, dreams, and myth. With the help of the maternal "reverie" it is possible for the infant to transform beta elements into alpha ones.

2. A passage from Bion comes to mind: "It is too often forgotten that the gift of speech, so centrally employed, has been elaborated as much for the purpose of concealing thought by dissimulation and lying as for the purpose of elucidating or communicating thought" (1970, p. 2).

3. W. Bion calls this maternal function "reverie." It describes the very special way in which a mother is connected empathically to her baby and is able to make sense of his communications, think about them in an affective way, and eventually name them.

4. Michael Fordham emphasized the relevance of the infant's personality and how this affects the relationship with the mother (Fordham 1967). Bion, on his part, wrote that "one circumstance that affects survival is the personality of the infant. Ordinarily, the personality of the infant, like other elements in the environment, is managed by the mother" (Bion 1967, p. 114).

References

Bion, W. 1967. *Second Thoughts*. London: Karnac, Meresfield, 1984.

———. 1970. *Attention and Interpretation*. London: Karnac, Meresfield, 1984.

Feldman, B. 1992. Jung's infancy and childhood and its influence upon the development of analytical psychology. *Journal of Analytical Psychology* 3,7:255–276.

Fordham, M. 1967. *Self and Autism*. London: Heinemann, Library of Analytical Psychology, 1976.

Jung, C. G. 1934. The soul and death. In *CW* 8:404–415. Princeton, N.J.: Princeton University Press, 1960.

———. 1968. *Memories, Dreams, Reflections*. London: Collins.

A Response to Mara Sidoli "Naming the Nameless"

Gareth S. Hill

Mara Sidoli has presented a very interesting paper, especially inso-far as it raises the issue of how we and our clients make sense of "no sense," what *kind* of sense is made of "no sense." This is what I would like to respond to in her paper, in the interest of stimulating discussion of some of the possible meanings to be found in the clinical material, how these meanings relate to one another, on the one hand, and how they might call for differing responses to the client, on the other hand.

I am mindful that, in this paper, Mara Sidoli strongly represents the school of analytical psychology built on the seminal work of Michael Fordham. By way of introduction, let me say that I am a member of the San Francisco institute where Fordham's school has long been sympa-thetically received by many of us and where, in the belief that dogma-tism is the shadow side of doubt, we pride ourselves on holding the tension between the clinical/developmental and the symbolic/synthetic approaches, appreciating the value and the necessity of each. Regarding this, in her paper "Transference and Countertransference," Ann Ulanov reminds us that

Gareth S. Hill is a Jungian analyst in private practice in Berkeley, California. He is on the faculty of the California Institute for Clinical Social Work, the Psychotherapy Institute of Berkeley, and the University of California at San Francisco. He is the author of *Masculine and Feminine: The Natural Flow of Opposites in the Psyche*.

Fordham correctly warns us against the tendency of patient and analyst alike to use the symbolic-synthetic perspective as a defense against uncovering the infantile roots of a complex. Jungians can easily waft themselves upwards into mythological spiritualizing, with talk about "the goddess" and "the gods," and thereby avoid the tough work involved in analyzing the anger that may be present in the transference, the envy, the sexual attraction, the embarrassment, and so on.

It is also fair to say that the fascinating work of exploring the early dynamic of introjected objects can be used as a defense against the pull of the archetype on the ego to get it out of placing itself, its wounds, its past, and its purposes at the center of the analytical experience. The product of this exaggeration is not a positive cooperation of ego and Self resulting in generosity to others, but rather an increasingly narrow and narcissistic concentration on the intricacies of the psychic process. (1982, p. 75)

We might begin by looking at the way young Andrew presented in the initial phase of his analysis. You will recall that, though he was very distressed and suicidal, for many sessions he kept up a matter-of-fact, cool, sophisticated conversation about education, literature, and theater, which were his hobbies, as if in a "literary salon," speaking rapidly without ever losing the stream of conversation. Actually, it sounds more like a monologue than a conversation, and Mrs. Sidoli understands it in a number of ways: she understands his speech as a way of concealing his distress and loneliness, his feelings of vulnerability and inferiority while making himself appear interesting and communicative; she understands it as a way of finding a connection with his mother who, he learned early, could only appreciate verbal communication; she understands his words as "autistic objects" to make himself feel alive, or as means of filling the gaps of time and space between them in order to protect himself from experiencing the analytic relationship as like his relationship with his mother—noncontaining, nonsoothing, and dead.

As I read Mrs. Sidoli's paper, I had a number of thoughts and associations, not different in their understanding of the fundamental underlying dynamic in this beginning analytic relationship, but with a different emphasis. Andrew appears to be compensating for feeling unsafe and untrusting in the treatment situation, which is unfamiliar to him, and he is terrified of the potential flow of his own authentic experience, which Mrs. Sidoli rightly sees him as having projected onto his girlfriend. In Jungian terms, Andrew is identified with persona, a learned adaptive response to maximize safety, security, and privacy in a new situation. In Henderson's terms, we might guess that Andrew is identified with a cultural attitude, apparently an aesthetic attitude and most likely his parents' cultural attitude, as a compensation for the terrifying absence of a secure sense of personal identity. In Winnicott's terms, Andrew reflects a false self that he has acquired in order to please and meet the expectations of the powerful adults in his life and to protect himself from the terror of their disapproval. In Kohut's terms, Andrew is in a merger transference; that is, he is so terrified of what he might find in the mirror of his analyst's regard that he can't bear for the mirror to be held up to him, he can't bear for her to be separate from him, different from him, to have a point of view of her own about him. He protects himself from the mirror by not letting her get a word in edgewise, by rendering her impotent, making it clear that he is not open to what she is making of what he is saying. All of these alternative views are ways of understanding essentially the same dynamic.

In this situation, the analyst faces the technical choice of working *with* the transference or *within* the transference, and Mrs. Sidoli isn't specific as to her approach. In my view, the wise choice is to take a position in a feminine mode of consciousness, in order to be as exquisitely attuned to and holding and containing of the client's experience as possible, in an effort to attract an archetypal transference. By archetypal transference, I mean a transference of those potentialities of the Self that are as yet unrealized in the client's experience. In this case, that would be the good, attuned, and affirming mother, the completely seen and understood child, and the trustworthy guide to the disorienting experience of psychic regression and transformation, which Andrew so far knows only in the tortured experience of his suicidal girlfriend. One would work within this developing archetypal transference until the client is assured that the treatment relationship is not dangerous to him. One would avoid any temptation to be the potent analyst who interprets the personal transference, because to do so could introduce an iatrogenic effect of prolonging the client's terror and mistrust. Although the personal transference interpretation may be technically correct, it does not address the client's immediate experience of the treatment situation in his own terms.

Mrs. Sidoli's paper doesn't reveal the vicissitudes of the treatment with regard to the developing therapeutic alliance. She does tell us of her needing to hold to her own thoughts during the early stages, which fits with my view of the wise choice of working within the transference. And her description of the quality of mothering that Andrew didn't have in his family situation is most moving, an understanding that supports the attraction of an archetypal transference of these potentialities. We also learn that, at some point, Andrew did move into suicidal behavior. In my experience, suicidal ideation is most likely to be concretized when there is doubt about the safety of the analytic container and about whether the analyst knows the way through the terror of regression. And further, although Mrs. Sidoli isn't specific with regard to the complexity of her theoretical orientation to this young man, much of her analysis of his relationship with her suggests a drive theory hypothesis, taking the emphasis away from the interactive and intersubjective dimensions of her understanding.

This is most aptly illustrated by the interpretation she makes about the damaged chair incident, the centerpiece of this case for the purposes of illustrating making sense of "no sense." She puts the emphasis upon his aggressive and destructive instinctual drives toward the mother in a genetic interpretation, which at first he resists. The interpretation touches something in him insofar as he palpably relaxes, but he appears unable to take in the intellectual substance of it. For me, this suggests that the interpretation was only partly experience-near. I would guess that it was experience-near insofar as it represented an acknowledgment from Mrs. Sidoli that something very important to Andrew had changed in the treatment situation. The content of the interpretation, however, appeared to be experience-distant, and Andrew resisted it. Mrs. Sidoli had made sense out of "no sense" for herself, but she may have presented Andrew with a "no sense" out of which he then had to make sense for himself.

I wondered what Andrew's response might have been had Mrs. Sidoli said in effect, "It has been difficult for you to feel comfortable and trusting in your relationship with me, and just as you are feeling that more, something that you have come to depend on is taken away from you, completely beyond your control." If there were an affective resonance from Andrew to an acknowledgment of what he faced in the immediate, concrete experience of their relationship, then the genetic elements in the chair mattering so much to him could perhaps have found a more experience-near resonance in Andrew. As it was, it took Andrew several sessions to acknowledge the content of the interpretation, and, perhaps unfairly, I was left with an uncertainty about the possible false self dimensions of his finally making sense of Mrs. Sidoli's "no sense." On this point, in a recent article called "Artist and Analyst," Philip Bromberg writes,

> The analyst . . . must be working with the patient in a way that . . . facilitates the patient's immediate experience of the analytic relationship as permitting

an evolving redefinition of the respective roles paralleling the patient's self growth. Only out of the creative use of such a context as "potential space" and the judicious exploration of its here-and-now evolution, can genetic interpretation and historical reconstruction aid in the integration of new self structure rather than global introjection of the analyst's "correct" interpretations. (1991, pp. 298–299)

Now let's turn to the dream of the second client, Linda. The dream was a complicated "no sense" of which Mrs. Sidoli and Linda made sense exclusively in terms of the personal family dimensions of Linda's life experience. In this regard, their work on the dream was impressive, highlighting the experience of the unseen, unacknowledged child in the pink satin dancing slippers, which represented her manic defense against experiencing her underlying depression and despair in the face of loss. It highlighted her frustrated need and rage about the deprivations in her life experience, but it also highlighted her being given an award for making it through the separation from Mrs. Sidoli. This latter seems to put emphasis on a transcendent factor in Linda's psychology that rewards her for relativizing her sufferings, moving the emphasis away from, as Ann Ulanov said, the ego's "placing itself, its wounds, its past, and its purposes at the center of the analytic experience."

This, in turn, brings an added significance to several decidedly nonpersonal, collective, if not archetypal elements in the dream that go unacknowledged by Mrs. Sidoli except at the personal level: namely, the aesthetic attitude, the four explosions, the flying, rocketlike synagogue, and the underlining of graffiti on bakery buildings. Let's be reminded that, though Linda was so very deprived of mother after age three, whatever the quality of mothering she had to that time, the mother archetype was strongly awakened in herself and provided her a means of survival, as manifested in her relationship to her brother and more recently in her relation to her work in which her mothering tendencies were quite out of control and threatening to her competence as a school counselor and budding psychotherapist. One might guess that there was far too little development of the masculine principle in Linda, and her relation to her spiritual life is also unexplored in Mrs. Sidoli's paper.

I think the nonpersonal images of the dream refer to these dimensions of her development and especially so in light of Linda entering her late middle years, in which the developmental task is to come to an objective realization of the sufferings of one's childhood as an aspect of one's fate that needs to be loved and needs to be appreciated as informing one's creative potentialities. The aesthetic perspective of Linda's artist friends relates to this. In their appreciation of the beauty in her adaptation to the necessity of leaving her attachment to her father and the sufferings of her childhood, they do appear to be denying of, or unmindful of, those sufferings, as Mrs. Sidoli points out. But, they are also appreciating the way in which her difficult separation-individuation out of her family informs her capacity for artistic expression, which she had long since denied in terms of being blocked from painting.

And what are we to make of the four explosions and the flying synagogue? We don't know whether Linda is Jewish or Gentile, but in either case, these powerfully energized images can be seen as references to the transpersonal Self, potentially dangerous, perhaps, because her relationship to this aspect of her development has been neglected. There is no longer any place to hide from it! Certainly, we Jungians would routinely view the number four as referring to Linda's potential wholeness, and in my view, it puts the emphasis on the neglected masculine aspect of the whole Self, the four points of the Christian cross, if you will; that is to say, the differentiated tension of opposites in an ordered state that would find expression in the capacity for boundaries, for finding security in appropriate structure rather than so singularly in attachment. And, the overwhelmingly energized image of a rocketlike flying synagogue also seems to me to have an obvious masculine referent. Certainly Linda needs to come to terms with Yahweh, the good and terrible Judaic god who is the author of bad things happening to good people, including innocent children. I particularly loved Linda underlining the graffiti on bakery buildings and her disgust with those who eat too many sweets. It appeared to be a collectively oriented image, perhaps a form of social protest. It reminded me that Britain has the highest per capita sugar consumption of any country in the world, as if a whole country is caught in an overreliance on this manifestation of the good breast. In any case, something in Linda appears to know that she has to protest and to overthrow this reality for the sake of her own development.

I would agree with Mrs. Sidoli's strategy of acknowledging and giving attention to the regressive aspects of Linda's psychic situation first, but I was troubled by the absence of any reference to the symbolic/synthetic dimension in making sense of the dream's "no sense." It is not that I would advocate directly interpreting these images along the lines I have suggested, but I think it is essential that the analyst consciously hold these amplifications so that they become a part of her total resonance to the client's unfolding development, informing the way she does relate to the client. I was frankly disturbed by the clinical implications of Linda's disordered behavior in throwing large stones at Mrs. Sidoli's garage door. It suggests to me that the regressive aspect of the work was overly concretized and literalized—that is, at that time at least, not treated as an essentially symbolic process that supports an appropriate adaptation to her sufferings of the reality of her life.

In conclusion, let me acknowledge that it is easy for the respondent to a short clinical presentation to second guess the work and find fault with it. That has not been my intention, because Mrs. Sidoli obviously has not been able to present much of the complexity and richness of her work with these patients over time in such a short paper. Rather, I hope to have used what she did present to focus for discussion some larger questions and issues about what we do and how we are as analysts.

References

Ulanov, A. 1982. Transference and countertransference. In *Jungian Analysis*, M. Stein, ed. La Salle, Ill.: Open Court.
Bromberg, P. 1991. Artist and analyst. *Contemporary Psychoanalysis* 27.

General Gordon's Constant Object

Fred Plaut

The person who is the subject of this paper had not been in analysis with me, for the most important reason that he died a violent death when he was slain at Khartoum in 1885, that is, before I was born and before there was any psychoanalysis. Less obviously, I can state without fear of contradiction that Charles George Gordon, fourth son of Henry William Gordon, born at Woolwich in 1833, is the only general in history to have proved to his entire satisfaction where the terrestrial paradise, the Garden of Eden, had been located and mapped it accordingly. This must do as a preliminary indication of Gordon's "eccentricity," as it was called in his day, before looking into the following questions, but not necessarily in strict order:

1. Why have I chosen a historical figure rather than a clinical case illustration?
2. Who was Gordon?
3. What is a constant object? What was Gordon's?
4. How does his mapping of paradise relate to madness?
5. What is the relation between psychopathology, madness, and Jung's concept of individuation?

Fred Plaut, M.B., B.Ch., D.P.M., is a training analyst and supervisor in private practice in Berlin. His previous publications include forty-two papers and contributions to four books. *Analysis Analyzed* is forthcoming from Routledge.

I think that the "mad parts" of a person dominate his or her true character. They attract our attention and are our bread and butter. If we can at all tolerate a person's madness, the person becomes both infuriating and endearing.

I shall not dwell long on the first question, as I do not feel guilty about having chosen a historical figure rather than a patient whose anonymity must be preserved. A biographic review is not the same as making direct analytical observations. But any report that is based on such direct observation, unique though it is, is also unavoidably colored by the analyst-reporter's theoretical spectacles and personal involvement. By contrast, the biographical portrait leading up the hero's death is like the unfolding of a drama on the stage. It, too, demands our participation, but our sense of personal responsibility is limited; what there is of it comes to us afterwards, mostly on reflection.

The less-involved observer of psychological phenomena has the onlooker's advantage of seeing most of the game in which he nevertheless participates. Of course, the near-total involvement or immersion of both partners is required to engender the necessary melting point at which the hoped-for transformations can occur. The changes expected are assumed to be changes for the better and to be lasting. But it is arguable that "better" is a very uncertain criterion, and we all know of relapses or of no fundamental changes having occurred. Neither Jung's nor Freud's most famous cases, Miss Miller and the Wolf Man, really changed. Miss Miller, whose case Jung had merely observed, in spite of all her symbols of transformation was readmitted to hospital. The Wolf Man, despite a second analysis with Freud and much analytically oriented therapy afterwards, remained recognizably the same patient.

Observing patients who do not change has led me to the conclusion that there is possibly a second kind of individuation inasmuch as the person becomes more and more himself or herself by way of their psychopathology or madness, their constant objects and preoccupations. It would be a travesty of what I mean by an alternative route if one were to conclude that every incurably mad person is or becomes for that very reason an individuated person. So allow me to clarify my position at the outset and to return to details later.

Hitherto our assumption has been that individuation could not proceed unless certain preconditions were fulfilled. The concept has been widened by both post-Jungians and psychoanalysts. Nevertheless, analysts have continued to assume that a certain state of development must necessarily precede individuation. That state is variously conceptualized as "integration," "object constancy," "symbolic attitude," or "union of opposites" and Klein's "depressive position." I am now going to argue, first, that individuation *can* develop not only in relation to but actually through a person's ordinary and unchanging psychopathology. The latter is seen as part of the self. And second, that the outcome of the individuation process cannot be judged in analytic terms only; sociocultural criteria must also be taken into consideration. To appreciate the significance of such criteria, let us proceed to the second question.

Who Was Gordon?

The present Gordon is, as I said, an analytical construct because the personal data available about his childhood are precious few. Sadly, we have no record of any dreams. Yet Gordon, who was in many ways a highly practical person, could, as we shall see, in other respects be called a dreamer. Trying to reconcile and make sense of the many puzzling features of Gordon's character has involved filling the gaps in the documentation with analytical speculations. Such speculations as I have ventured are, nevertheless, deduced from my wider analytical knowledge of persons with comparable characteristics who I have known as patients or in a social context and from biographies. As analysts, we are used to attaching a great deal of importance to the developmental history and are forever on the alert for clues which could help us make links with later developments. As early clues are scarce here, it is likely that I have given undue weight to such descriptions as we do have of Gordon's personality and character. It so happens that we know more about Gordon of Khartoum than we know of Charlie Gordon as he was known to family and friends. Although far from being wholly fictitious, I must stress that my Gordon has nevertheless been constructed with the psychopathology of constant objects, madness, and individuation in mind. But then, most "case reports" are also the outcome of similar constructions reflecting the mind of the writer as much as that of the patient.

When the haze of hero worship which followed his death had dispersed, there remained an unusual and, in many ways, admirable as well as complex and tragic character.

He started his brilliant military career as "Chinese" Gordon (because of his outstanding military leadership during the Taiping rebellion) and ended it as "Gordon of Khartoum" (the city he refused to surrender). When he was sent to evacuate Khartoum, it was clear to those who knew him that the decision would end in combat, and sure enough, not only was the city besieged, but a tragedy unfolded as the *dramatis personae* confronted each other. The Mahdi was no less a convinced Moslem than Gordon was a Christian, and both, in their way, were noble warriors. Impulsive and hasty activity by Gordon was opposed by delay in organizing an expeditionary force to raise the siege. On January 28, 1885 (it would have been his fifty-second birthday), the relief column arrived. Gordon had been killed and subsequently decapitated two days earlier.

Is it as a hero who chose death rather than surrender his Christian faith or abandon his post that Gordon remains an impressive and fascinating figure? Certainly this interpretation was current at the time (twenty-five books were written about him in the first eighteen months after his death), and it strikes a sufficiently archetypal note to account for the nationwide mourning and worship that followed. But Gordon had courted death, and his behavior at Khartoum was perfectly in keeping with his personality.

A man of remarkable integrity and fearlessness, Gordon was often very awkward to deal with and was widely regarded as "eccentric," even a little crazy.

One biographer, Nutting, entitled his book *Gordon: Martyr and Misfit* (1966). Gordon constantly quarreled with authority, to the point of disobeying orders, and his tendency toward asceticism was certainly not shared by his Victorian contemporaries. Who else would have slashed his own salary, as Governor-General of the Sudan, from 10,000 to 2,000? "I am," he wrote, "like Moses who despised the riches of Egypt . . ." The Chinese, too, became decidedly anxious when he refused to take their bribes.

He suffered furious outbursts of temper, often followed by complete withdrawal—cutting off all contact, reading the Bible, and drinking cognac. Yet he was never seen to be the worse for drink. His tendency to self-criticism and remorse was considerable: when he emerged from his self-imposed isolation, he was at pains to make amends to those he had hurt or punished. Indifferent to physical hardship, he could also long to lie in bed until eleven every day and eat oysters ("not a dozen but four dozen"). More than once he gave up alcohol and tobacco: it was a running battle between making a pledge and yielding to temptation. Yet, despite his unpredictable moods, all descriptions of him agree that he appeared to have been happy most of the time, goodhumored and full of energy.

Quite the most important aspects of his character are his version of religion and his sexual orientation. What are the details?

Gordon, in accordance with the ideal of the times, but unlike most Victorians of his class, lived simply and gave generously to those in need. Abstinence was a virtue and death the ultimate triumph of the spirit over the flesh: the dichotomy between the flesh and the spirit was, for him, absolute. Death was to be wished for devoutly, yet to hasten it would be sinful, for God had given us work to do — was this the reason why he was fearless in the face of physical danger?

As to Gordon's sexuality, it seems well attested that he was more homosexual than heterosexual. He avoided opportunities to meet eligible ladies, said that marriage was not for him, and befriended young boys. It is improbable that he was ever a practicing homosexual; in a man who lived so much in the public eye and had many enemies, this could hardly have escaped notice. The public view of his time was that a man could do without sex or amuse himself from time to time with those ladies whose profession it was. Of course, there is no evidence to that effect either; but, no doubt, he suffered. At the age of fifty, in a letter to a friend, the Reverend R. H. Barnes, he wrote, "I wished I was a eunuch at fourteen . . ."

In his family history, there are no more than a few pointers to Gordon's development other than his having been a mischievous boy, remarkable also for his "high spirits and pluck" as one biographer (Strachey 1918) had remarked. A later biographer referred to these characteristics as "naughty, ruthless and resourceful" (Trench 1978). Charlie was sent to boarding school (Taunton) at the age of nine, where he did not distinguish himself except for his skill in drawing maps. His father was of Highland and military descent and had risen to the rank of Lieutenant General, Royal Artillery, a rank which our Gordon never achieved. His mother came from a family of merchants, well known for their sea voyages. Charlie was the fourth son of eleven children and had been destined for the Royal Artillery. But owing to an act of uncontrolled temper and near insubordination, there was a delay in the officer-cadet being commissioned and so he went into the Royal Engineers. What data we have are from his adult life, when he found his mother demanding and possessive after his father's death. This occurred in 1865, when Gordon was thirty-two, and he dated his religious conversion to that year. Earlier, however, a mild dose of smallpox in China had made him reflect on things eternal: "I am glad to say," he wrote to his sister Augusta (a formidable spinster with whom he shared his theological theories in a long and voluminous correspondence), "that the disease has brought me back to my Saviour." Although Gordon had shown no religious inclinations as a boy and never joined any church nor was confirmed, he seems to have come under the evangelist and salvationist influence of a Captain Drew when he was staying at Pembroke, where he took the first sacrament at Easter 1854 when he was twenty-one. He also began to study the Bible, examining every passage minutely to discover the true meaning with results that seemed extraordinary to other people. We note that Gordon dates his conversion to the year his father died. Actually the conversion seems to have taken place some ten years earlier, after he met Drew. Later we shall refer to the special purifying role that communion had in Gordon's religious view.

Although Gordon passionately believed that what distinguished Christianity from all other religions was God's indwelling in man, a condition was attached: belief in Jesus as God the Son. He printed and distributed his own religious tracts, embarrassing complete strangers with queries as to the state of their faith, and his constant Bible reading led him to speculation far beyond what would be regarded as normal for a Christian living in the Victorian era. He determined where Satan would finally be imprisoned—in the center of the earth, having been sucked down through the Dead Sea. Similarly, he decided where Our Lord now was: "Being a Man He must be in some definite place" (see chapter in Trench, *Reflections in Palestine*). He concluded that Christ was hovering just over Jerusalem, above the altar of the true temple. "All prayer (from whatever part of the globe) must pass by and through Him . . ." To a modern reader, this might provoke comparison with a communications satellite, but for Gordon there was no "as if" about this or anything else. If the Lord and Satan were real, they must have HQs and these had to be properly located.

The Discovery of Eden

In 1881, languishing on leave in England (one of his periodic resignations from the Army having been refused), Gordon met a friend, Colonel Sir Howard Elphinstone, who lamented having been posted to Mauritius, a terrible backwater for a Royal Engineer. Gordon offered to take Elphinstone's place; this was accepted, and he left England shortly afterwards. From a letter to "My dear Elphin," we gather that Gordon may have regretted his generosity. However, once in Mauritius, he took up his Bible studies again and also became interested in botany. The combination was important for what was to follow, for Gordon, receiving orders to look into the harbor installations on Mahé, the largest of the Seychelles, also visited the neighboring island, Praslin, which he promptly identified as the site of the vanished Garden of Eden.

Praslin is the only place in the world where a palm tree grows which bears that strange fruit, the *coco de mer*. Gordon describes "its fruit shaped in the husk like a heart, when opened like a belly with thighs." I am quoting from a manuscript in my possession entitled *"Eden and Its Two Sacramental Trees"*; it consists of eight folio pages in Gordon's writing, accompanied by two pages of maps in color; it is signed by him and dated 26.2.82.

Charles Chenevix Trench (1978) tells us that Gordon's theory was based on "the remarkable similarity between the ripe fruit of the *coco de mer* a gigantic palm tree, and Eve's pudenda" (p. 171). Delicately put . . . and no one who sees the illustrations, including Gordon's photograph of the fruit, could mistake what he means. We know that his friend Gessi, possibly with reference to the photograph, said: "Carlo has never seen what there is between a woman's legs" (MacGregor-Hastie 1985, p. 143). Certainly Gordon was in no doubt that this was the fruit from the Tree of Knowledge (figure 1).

The *coco de mer (Lodoicea seychellarum)* had occasionally been washed ashore in India and Africa. Before Praslin was discovered to be its original home, it was thought to grow at the bottom of the sea. Numerous legends surround it, including the not unlikely story that the Holy Roman Emperor, Rudolf II, had offered 4,000 florins for one of the fruits because it was reputed to be an antidote to poison. A tale survives to this day that the semitransparent, glutinous pulp (which makes good eating either as a fruit or as a vegetable) has "other invigorating qualities."

Although it is called a double coconut, this is, according to botanists, a misnomer. What matters, however, is that there is a male and a female tree — and no difficulty in distinguishing between the two (figure 2). One writer describes the male tree as being covered here and there with groups of phalli, each about eighteen inches to two feet long and three or four inches in diameter. It is said that these become erectile after sunset and remain so until sunrise.

In another remarkable palm tree (the breadfruit, *Artocarpus incisa*), Gordon recognized the Tree of Life. So there on Praslin were the trees, the climate was right, and "there was also a 3-foot long serpent there," Gordon adds.

It is the second part of Gordon's essay that is devoted to the sacramental trees, and the opening sentence of these pages reads:

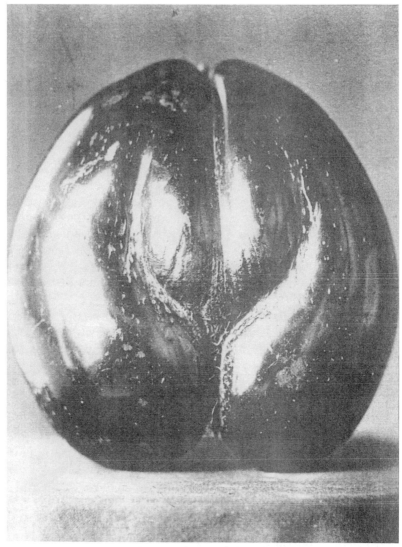

Figure 1. The *coco de mer*, Gordon's photograph.

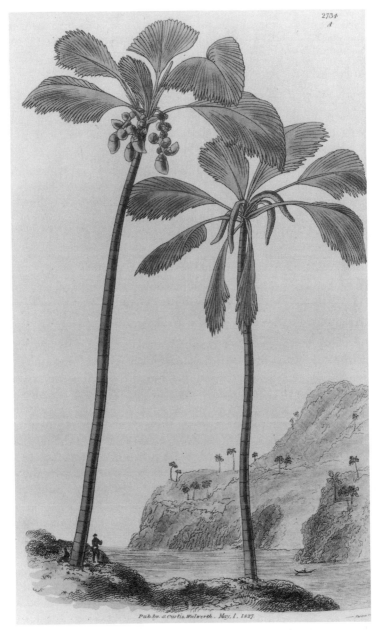

Figure 2. The male and female trees.

> God has used instruments at all ages, to manifest Himself to man, these
> instruments though nothing in themselves, were everything when connected
> with Him. (Gordon 1882, p. 5)

Gordon gives a few examples showing that

> when things are done with, they pass back, are relegated into ordinary
> things. . . thus there is no reason why the two trees which were in the Garden
> of Eden should not exist to this day. They fulfilled their functions and are
> relegated back to their ordinary condition. The bread and wine in themselves
> are nothing yet they are Christ's flesh and blood.

(We note he uses "are," not "symbolize.") Gordon's explanation for the
dual nature or state of being is in keeping with his dichotomy between
the flesh and the spirit, and these are accompanied by a more elementary one, between *male* and *female*. After the "belly and thighs" comparison, he continues:

> It is a magnificent tree, the Prince of trees in every way and full of types, its
> germination is extraordinary when taken with the words ye generation of
> serpents.

> "O generation of vipers, who hath warned ye to flee from the wrath to come?
> Bring forth therefore fruits meet for repentence." (Matthew 3, 78)

The point here is that "the tree of knowledge" is not hermaphroditic
like the coconut palm but is divided into two sexes. Gordon's "types"
look as if they foreshadowed the "Fall" by virtue of this sexual differentiation and germination—they represent the forbidden knowledge on a
botanical level (see figures 3a and 3b). Like the other objects which he
enumerates as examples of ordinary things, the "extraordinary" germination was apparently all right, since when "God used them, they were
most holy" (Gordon 1882, p. 5). Yet Gordon never succeeded in
accepting the union of opposite sexes, even as a necessity for the propa-
gation of mankind, although the requisite parts were being, or could
be regarded as being, used by God.

Trench quotes the correspondence between Gordon and W. Scott
(superintendent of the Royal Botanical Garden at Pamplemousses)
which includes anatomical sketches by Gordon of Eve's reproductive
system. Gordon wanted to know whether the flower of the breadfruit
(his Tree of Life) were male, female, or hermaphrodite. Would Scott
put him in touch with the Liverpool doctor who had examined a pregnant man? Sexual confusion, sexual differentiation, and union—and,
above all, the search for a way in which union could be made comprehensible and therefore innocuous to the soul—seem to have been the
mainspring behind Gordon's curiosity.

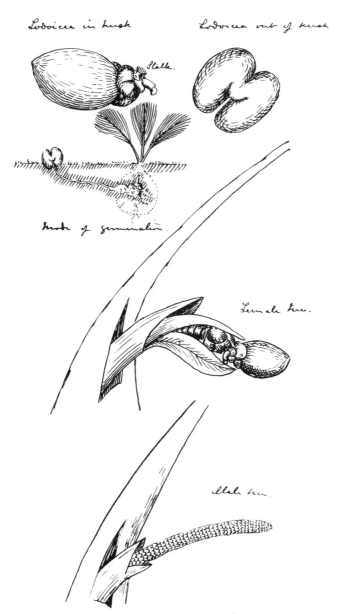

Figure 3a. Details of the *coco de mer*.

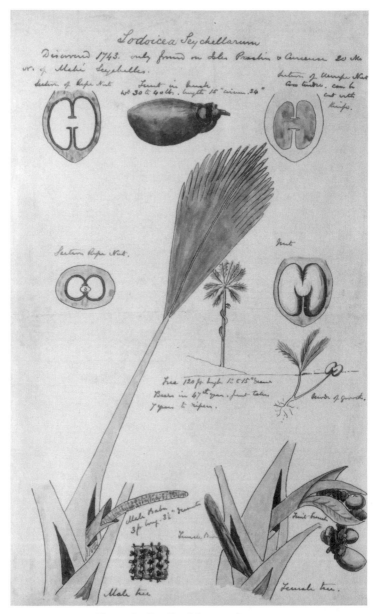

Figure 3b. Details of the *coco de mer*.

Gordon needed a reconciling symbol, and the illustrations make it understandable that the sight of the forbidden fruit of the *coco de mer* displaced the authenticity of the humble but traditional paradisical apple. When he had "pretty well settled the site of Eden, of the Garden and the Trees of Knowledge and Life" (letter to Augusta), he rejoiced that "Milton wonderfully works it into my idea," (Trench 1978, p. 172) and quotes from *Paradise Lost* (Book IV, 1.218):

> And all amid them stood the tree of Life
> High eminent, blooming ambrosial fruit
> of vegetable gold

Milton (though not Gordon) continues the line as follows:

> and next to life,
> our death, the Tree of Knowledge, grew fast by
> Knowledge of good, bought dear by knowing ill.

The omission is significant. Gordon never forgave Eve, or accepted the Fall as a necessary evil, and he selected from Milton's poem only those lines which he regarded as confirmatory evidence for his topographical discovery. But Milton's description was poetic and symbolical, not to be used as a guidebook, as Gordon seems to do. Gordon then expatiates on the sequence of events in the Garden:

> Adam (and Eve) were perfectly free from any temptation except that of eating of the Tree of Knowledge. Luxury, power, etc., etc., which are temptations to man now could have no effect on these two, the only way they could be tempted was by their stomachs and by curiosity. (1882, pp. 67)

> They ate and they fell. Now I believe that neither had the very faintest idea of what would follow, that their act was one we commit every moment, as to say forgetting God and trusting self, heedlessness, greediness, forgetfulness. They were poisoned, and I must say that I think, if it is looked deeply into, there is a close analogy between the first eating and the second eating of Christ's Body and Blood. By the first eating we commune with Satan, by the second eating we commune with [illegibile word in MS] Christ. (Ibid., p. 7)

Here Gordon is traveling a well-worn path, reminiscent of his pamphlet, issued in earlier years, entitled "Take Eat." Christ's injunction "Do this in remembrance of me" (the words accompanying the communion) are then repeated, and the tone of the manuscript becomes admonishing and preaching:

> We shall never get power over our bodies till we take the antidote of the poison we have in us, a child can understand you have eaten what does make you ill, eat this for your cure. (Ibid., p. 8)

A little later, he castigates Eve (without excusing Adam or accusing Satan):

> What did Eve think, did she go and study the tree, no, she took and ate to see for herself, she wanted to gratify herself . . . (Ibid.)

Obviously he saw no connection between Eve's lapse and his own insubordinations and episodic incontinence—his rages, drinking, and excessive smoking. Although for secular occasions he relied on self-control or willpower (Richard Burton, the African explorer, noted Gordon's "controul"), he could not escape his obsession. The flesh *must* be defeated by the spirit. The only antidote to the Tree of Knowledge, from which springs sexuality, is the second eating, the sacrament of the communion. The bread and wine become the means or instruments by which we are purified of willful disobedience.

There are a number of extraordinary contradictions in all this. First, Gordon's conflict—between wanting to do good and be abstemious on the one hand, and his inclination to contrariness on the other—finds its remedy in the communion and, generally, in trying to follow Christ. He believes in that antidote literally: *not by transubstantiation, but as if it consisted of minute particles* descending from Heaven. Similarly, he regards the attributes of evil as having been physically introduced into Eve's body: "the fruit was the vehicle of *the virus of evil*" (and he does not use this phrase as a mere metaphor).

Second, while the Fall is brought about by temptation (via the stomach), it introduces sexual knowledge. And for Gordon, there appears to be no sacrament, such as marriage, which will counteract that poison. Eve cannot become "the means" or instrument by which God works.

Gordon seems to have forgotten that Jesus, the son of Man, was thereby also a descendant of Eve, albeit with the addition of special purifications (the immaculate conception, the virgin birth). Milton summed it up by writing about the Messiah: "So God with man unites . . ." Not for Gordon these glad tidings. Eve, and thereby Man, remains *unredeemed during her lifetime*, except for occasional dispensations by means of the antidote.

The manuscript ends on a note of modified pessimism:

> The two trees are here now, and we eat daily sometimes of one, sometimes (less frequently) of the other the tree of life. In return, the tree of knowledge is

dying out, men have eaten it nearly up, its effects are manifest, the tree of life shall exist more abundantly, but few eat of it, except the poor. The table of the Lord is contemptible not worth considering. *Mal*. 1.7. (Ibid. p. 8)

The final statement contradicts the earlier assertion, namely, the return to the ordinary state of things after God has made use of them. *Their instrumentality persists* in a negative way when Gordon requires it to serve as a dire warning, no doubt as much to himself as to those he wanted to address, and God's "union with man" via Eve and the Virgin is denied. No reconciling symbol for Gordon.

Gordon had been stimulated by the sight of the "forbidden fruit," the *coco de mer* — and his ideas, intuitions, and rationalizations did the rest, finding expression in the manuscript and the accompanying maps. The major driving force for his extraordinary theories seems to be the return to a conflict-free state, prior to temptation — to be a eunuch at fourteen . . . to be dead. His literal, childlike comprehension of the Bible — and his apparent inability to grasp symbolic meanings — helps us to understand his longing to return to the Garden of Eden as it was before the Fall.

Gordon's Map and the Rivers of Eden

The opening sentence of "Eden and Its Two Sacramental Trees" reads, "God works by means and by natural laws." (The phrase "by means" — according to the Shorter O.E.D. — refers to the resources, but also to the *instrumentality*, of things or persons.) And so I have deliberately postponed discussion of the first part of Gordon's manuscript, because the inspiration for the search, the means or instrumentality, should come before "the natural laws."

Gordon used his knowledge of these laws in order to rationalize what he intuited after seeing the *coco de mer*. His geographical and geological arguments, if one can call them that, certainly strain credulity where he relies for supportive evidence on the Bible and on etymology. But when he proceeds to account for the four rivers of Eden, his knowledge as a Royal Engineer is harnessed in support of his thesis, and this is where we meet the working of his mind in its most original and ingenious, but also eccentric, productivity. For the lengths to which he had to go to make the rivers flow to his location are nothing short of extraordinary.

The first logical step for anyone taking Genesis as his guidebook is to reconstruct the world as it was before the Flood — and Gordon makes us imagine, with the help of an illustration, the way the rivers flowed at

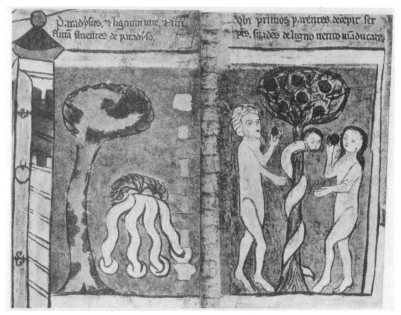

Figure 4. Medieval representation of paradise detail in
Ebstorf map.

that time. He stipulates a habitable zone or belt around the equator,
toward which (before the earth was tilted on its axis) all rivers from the
melting northern and southern icecaps flowed. When God's breath, in
the form of fire, produced the Flood, it caused the toppling over by
23 $1/2°$ of the upper northern hemisphere (because of its greater land
mass, it carried more ice than the lower hemisphere). Floods do not
change the general features of land, but simply modify them by silting
up rivers in low-lying land, or blocking up channels and causing rivers
to change their course.

Gordon writes:

> To the Rev. Berry I owe the final thought on the subject of the site of Eden. I
> had already thought that the two trees were distinguishable at Seychelles.
> (1882, p. 2)

He now reverses the usual interpretation of Genesis, that a river flowing
from Eden watered the Garden and then branched into four streams, as
"the mass of men" falsely believe (see figure 4). But Gordon, with the

help of the Rev. D. Berry, translates this not as "four rivers" (or streams) but as "four heads" (i.e., origins), which form one great antediluvian river basin:

> in no instance in this world do we find four rivers flowing out of one river, while there are many instances of four rivers flowing into one. (Ibid.)

This is the geological basis from which Gordon launches a hypothesis which becomes more and more bizarre as he continues. He states that west of the Seychelles there is a deep basin in the Indian Ocean (see figure 5). (This is correct: it has a depth of 2,600 fathoms.) He mentions a cleft near Socotra which has two branches, one of which runs up the Persian Gulf, the other up the Red Sea. (I have not been able to trace these "branches" from the information likely to have been available to Gordon, and modern oceanography does not confirm their existence.)

The Tigris, having been joined by the Euphrates, comes down the Persian Gulf and forms the eastern branch. "We have therefore two rivers we want two more" writes Gordon (p. 3), clinging fast to elementary arithmetic.

The remaining two rivers are called "Pison" and "Gihon" in Genesis. While other reconstructions regard the Gihon as the Nile and the Pison as the Indus or Ganges, Gordon's, not surprisingly, does the opposite. He admits that we have no very clear clue to these two, but as Babylon and Nineveh, situated on the banks of the Euphrates and the Tigris, were opponents of Israel, "so the other two rivers we want must have this peculiarity also."

Whatever the truth of the matter, it would be difficult to find a better example of how misleading an argument by analogy can be. By a variety of attributes, other than Egypt's enmity to Israel, Gordon proves to his satisfaction that the Pison is the Nile.

> The Nile is considered by good authorities to have once discharged into the Red Sea and its changing its course after the Flood is not a very improbable thing as the land is low and much silt must have swept down with the melting glaciers.

The Canal of Hero appears as a dotted line on Gordon's map; although not lettered as such, his brother, H. W. Gordon, in his biography makes this explicit. Hero was an Alexandrian mathematician and inventor who lived ca. 250 B.C.; the canal connected the Nile north of Suez with Lake Timsah and hence the Red Sea. The anachronism of the antediluvian situation represented in Gordon's map is obvious, for the Flood predated the Canal.

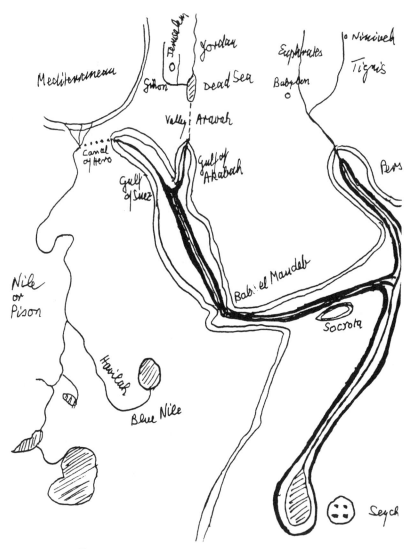

Figure 5. Gordon's map of the site of Eden (copied by author).

"The Gihon is the next river," but its course proves even trickier than the Pison's. Gordon identifies the Gihon in the now dried-out riverbed or brook just south of Jerusalem which by a deep ravine falls via the Valley of Fire into the Dead Sea. As for the common denominator, the opponent of Israel, he writes:

In Genesis [2:13] Gihon is said to encompass the land of Cush. Cush was the son of Nimrod and Nimrod was of Assyria.

In the sentence which follows, Gordon finds a rather confused way of regarding genealogy and hereditary enmity as more important than the historical geography which usually equates the land of Cush with Ethiopia. He simply reiterates: "I therefore think the Gihon [in the vicinity of Jerusalem] is the Gihon of Eden." There remains the difficulty of bringing Gordon's Gihon from the Dead Sea into the Red Sea, but this is overcome (in the main) by means of an underground river (see figure 6).

The rest is smooth sailing. The cleft coming from the Red Sea carries the waters of both Pison (Gordon's Nile) from Suez and Gihon from the Gulf of Akaba. It flows via Aden. "Aden is Eden," writes Gordon. What could be more obvious? For "Eden was a district [i.e., in what is now the Indian Ocean], the Garden of Eden was a chosen spot." The antediluvian riverbeds joined northeast of the Island of Socotra, and from there the great river flowed south-by-west to water the Garden of Eden. To make all this "real" and thereby convincing, Gordon illustrates his thesis by skillfully drawn and sometimes colored maps.

Gordon Among the Paradise Mappers

Gordon's talent for drawing maps had been noted at school: his letters are interspersed with elegant botanical or zoological sketches and illustrative maps. But it is chiefly Gordon's idiosyncrasies which give him a unique place among modern cartographical reconstructions, for although he may have been aware of other attempts in modern times to locate the site of Eden, there is no indication that he had the slightest idea that he was following in the footsteps of Christian cartographers going as far back as the sixth century A.D. What are the reasons for this remarkable regress? Such is the complexity of historical and psychological factors that a classification, however rough, is required to provide a perspective and a background against which Gordon's attempt to put the Garden of Eden on the map must be viewed.

The attempt to bring Gordon's map into the context of other mappers of paradise will bring a principle into focus which has received

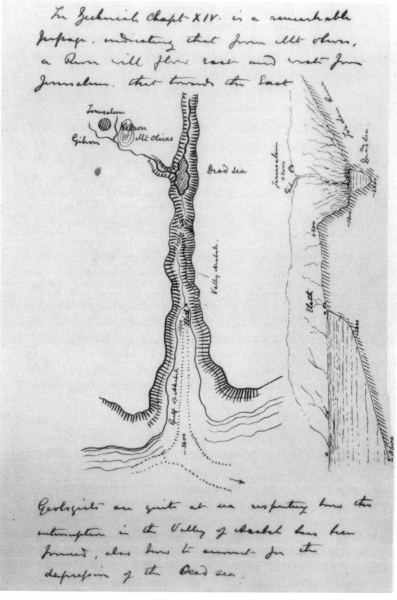

Figure 6. Gordon's Gihon.

insufficient attention in analytical circles. Analysis being a specialized subject, has, like other specialities, tacitly assumed that its findings are of equal importance in all parts of the world and at all times; or, alternatively, that archetypal patterns are invariant, only their mode of expression changes. I find this generalization too sweeping. *It leaves out the cultural dimension as an important factor in the conduct as well as in the retrospective evaluation of a person's life.* In Gordon's case, this meant the Victorian era, the height of the empire, and his having been a member of a distinct social class. The present example shows that what must be regarded as "pathological," abnormal, eccentric, or even psychotic in our time, would have been perfectly in keeping with the worldview (*Weltanschauung*) of another age. One might well wonder whether Gordon, had he lived today, would have become the subject of as much hero worship as he did in the Victorian era, at the height of the British empire. As an eccentric character he was, no doubt, a nuisance to officialdom and treated accordingly. Dying as he did would have aroused sympathy at any time. But hero worship at a time when the country was not at war? It seems more than doubtful.

My going into detail about Gordon's mapping of Eden is meant to demonstrate the relationship between the historical and cultural setting and the way an individual's action and character are psychologically assessed. In doing so I hope to make an addition to the criteria by which we may distinguish an abortive or pathological form of individuation from the virtual goal of personality development that Jung has proposed.

But to return to Gordon. Had he lived at the time of Cosmas Indico Pleustes, an Alexandrian monk who lived and traveled in the sixth century, his attempt to map Eden and other biblical localities would not have aroused the suspicion of his being a crank or worse. On the contrary, it would have earned him the approval of faithful souls who regarded biblical authority as the ultimate source of truth. Indeed, he would have added to their faith the dimension which we, in our time, regard with equal confidence as unquestionable, namely scientific evidence. Gordon's arguments are, for us, pseudoscientific and as absurd as Cosmas's, who in his *Topographia Christiana* showed the world shaped in the form of the tabernacle with Eden as a separate oblong part in the east beyond the ocean. Although Cosmas's successors deviated from his tenet by mapping the world in the shape of a disc, Cosmas's localization of Eden and its four rivers in the east remained the authoritative cartographical model.

With the advent of the Renaissance and the age of discoveries, the location of paradise on the map became doubtful and therefore mobile. That is to say, the existence of the cradle of mankind as a geographical place was not in doubt. But now there were rival theories regarding its exact whereabouts. "In the East" was no longer precise enough. That it was a zone into which reentry had been forbidden no longer deterred explorers from inventing rival theories. One of these, a sea chart from the fifteenth century, places the Garden fairly close to Gordon's Seychelles, namely in east Africa. Gradually, however, Eden became extruded from the body of the map and was awarded an honorable place as a marginal decorative detail. The mapmaker himself may have had doubts, but he played it safe and satisfied the customer.

A further stage in paradise mapping was reached in modern times when variously motivated persons reconstructed the site. Gordon was not the last person so to do. But his thesis is as bizarre as von Wendrin's, who, motivated by antisemitism, resited paradise in 1924 between northern German provinces. Gordon, being the person he was, reconstructed the site in an unusual place much further south than east of Jerusalem. In 1919, Sir William Willcocks, a British water engineer, came to the conclusion that the Garden had been situated in Mesopotamia. A more plausible location, it is true, and one that was in keeping with Genesis and the Bible maps of the sixteenth to eighteenth centuries. But what is it that makes a person in modern times want to find a geographical site for a symbolic image at all? We shall have to return to the question, using what we know about Gordon in order to understand the phenomenon analytically (see "Literal Mindedness" below).

Gordon in Context

Placing Gordon among the mappers of paradise both ancient and modern gives the text a historical and cultural context, a dimension of which analysis takes insufficient notice. Whereas in past centuries the mapping of paradise was quite common and perfectly in keeping with the prevailing implicit faith in revealed biblical knowledge, reconstruction of the site of the Garden had become in Gordon's time an anachronistic phenomenon requiring the particular outlook referred to in the text. Had he lived two hundred years earlier, Gordon's mapping of paradise would, as we saw, have been in keeping with the tradition of literal Bible interpretation. Only the spot he had chosen would have caused criticism. In a still earlier century, at the time of Calvin, he would have been accused of heresy with the usual dire consequences.

Not that this would have deterred Gordon. In fact, it would have suited him quite well, as we shall presently see.

But taken by itself, literal mindedness does not explain why a colonel of the Royal Engineers should, in the course of his duties, have linked a series of diverse and dubious facts in order to construe and actually map the site of the biblical place. Living in the post-Darwinian era, most educated persons would have regarded Eden as a symbolical reference to humankind's origin. As part of a cosmogenic myth, the location of paradise is irrelevant. To map it was an anachronism. The mapper's state of mind would therefore be in doubt; why should he wish to turn the clock back? Gordon did not see it that way.

From a biographer's point of view, Gordon's affair with Eden was not an important milestone. Whether it was passed over with politeness or embarrassment, the "discovery" seems to have received no attention. But psychologically, the illustrated essay epitomizes its author's repeated preoccupation with a combination of sexual and religious matters. What made Gordon's brand of religion highly idiosyncratic was, as we saw, the mixture of literal mindedness and salvationism. From our point of view, Gordon's "constant object" was his God. Unlike Job, however, Gordon never questioned but idealized God, just as he demonized Satan and his instruments, foremost the "flesh" in the form of Eve.

But let us first turn to the social and cultural milieu, without which no one can be understood. There were eleven siblings in all, of which Charlie was the fourth son. Nothing unusual seems to have occurred during his mother's pregnancy nor at birth. The circumstances as well as the exposure to daily Bible readings from an early age were perfectly standard features considering the family's social background and the Victorian era. We also know that his family had moved house about half a dozen times before he was nine, when he was sent to boarding school.

We can assume that despite having so many children on her hands, Elizabeth Gordon managed to give enough care to all so that none of them died, as frequently happened in those days. Whether each of them received the special personal attention that, from today's point of view, they required is improbable. The parents did not neglect their marital and social duties on account of the large household in which Bible readings were supplemented by the large collection of religious tracts in Elizabeth Gordon's hands. Nothing suggests that fairy tales were ever read to the children. Nor did poetry or music figure in the home. One can be fairly sure that their conscience was more frequently catered to than their imagination. All this appears quite up to the standard accepted for the bringing up of children at the time. We must therefore question whether whatever it was that made Gordon the highly unique person he was as well as an "eminent Victorian" was due to specific environmental influences. This question is all the more cogent when we know of no unusual or exceptional features in his ten siblings. It seems more likely that his constitution including gifts, sensitivity, and homosexual leaning led to a specific reaction to or against a "normal" family life. This it was more than anything else that made him an individual and caused his suffering. Officialdom did the rest.

Gordon's Constant Object

Psychopathology, Madness and, Possibly, Individuation

In my contributing chapter to *Psychopathology: Contemporary Jungian Perspectives* (1991), I went into detail about the concept of object constancy. Now I shall try to recapitulate and condense the characteristics of a constant object which are most relevant to our case and to which I already referred at the outset. It will help us to differentiate between the *merely mad* and the *also mad but apparently sane* person if we bear in mind that the path of object constancy requires the person's ability to appreciate symbolically that opposite characteristics can emanate from one and the same object to which the ego relates. For some people, this is too difficult to ever appreciate; others manage it some of time, and nobody all the time. As the difference between the constant object about which I am writing here and the much better known object constancy is crucial, I shall summarize the terms used by analytical schools which, for practical purposes, are equivalent.

1. We have *ambivalence,* which is engendered by conflict; the underlying contradictory emotional attitudes such as love and hate can be recognized as coming from the same source. A realistic assessment of the imperfect nature of an object becomes possible with ambivalence (Rycroft 1968).
2. The term *object constancy* indicates a further development. It was probably coined by Hartmann and used by the American school of ego psychology (Hartmann 1964, pp. 163, 173). The term refers to the ability to maintain lasting relationships with a single object for which substitutes are rejected. The object's

identity and that of the ego are seen to merge in object constancy.

3. Melanie Klein's *depressive position* indicates the developmental phase in which ambivalence can develop out of the previous phase, which she calls the paranoid-schizoid position. The important point is that the depressive position is not attained once and for all and regression to the previous phase can and does occur throughout life.

4. Finally there are terms with which we, as Jungians, are familiar, particularly in terms of symbol formation. They are referred to as "union of opposites" and in practice also as "holding the opposites together."

No matter what terms we employ in our work, patience is clearly indicated. As Jung writes, in "The Stages of Life": "The meaning and purpose of a problem seem to lie not in its solution but in our working at it incessantly" (1931, par. 771). What really matters to me is whether analysts can keep an open mind toward those patients whose capacity to develop along the path of object constancy is severely limited. Given some talent such patients may have for expressing their devotion to a constantly good and even idealized object, they may nevertheless lead satisfying lives. For them, the alternative, which I called the constant object, may be therapeutic, as I outlined in my earlier paper under the subheading, "Devotion versus Addiction" (Plaut 1974). The dangers of inflation, paranoia, and depression are just as great with the alternative route to individuation as they are with the classical kind. Therefore, a relatively constant object, even if it is derived from and bears the hallmarks of a cult object, is a valuable and necessary standby. This can serve as a focal point for a personality that would otherwise be in danger of disintegration. Provided only that the ego does not become totally absorbed by it, the constant object offers the person a viable alternative, a chance to integrate around an alternative core. What I think saved Gordon from becoming totally mad and fanatical was his astonishing degree of tolerance of persons of other races and religious persuasions. This is a quality which is not always found among analysts who know all about images of wholeness and union of opposites. The object which I call constant here is Gordon's "God" or his representative to God-Man, Jesus. It demands a constancy or persistence of the believer's faith in his object. If he falters, he sins. What made his "begoddedness" so essential was the repression of sexuality, and of homosexuality in particular. The extraordinary expression of the constant object in the form of a paradise map was conditioned by what I shall refer to as literal mindedness or asymbolia. In psychoanalytic terms, this inflexibility may be psychopathological and would be referred to as repetition compulsion, meaning the tendency not to change or to revert to earlier states of mind. The tendency is regarded as innate. Therefore, the term can only *describe* a psychic condition, but it doesn't explain it psychodynamically. It is nevertheless used as if it were a way to explain resistance to therapeutic change (See Rycroft 1968). In analysis, repetition compulsion is something that the patient is expected to "give up."

It would be true to say that Gordon's essay, the core of our text, bristles with clues to his unchanging psychopathology. Therefore, we must ask what the most outstanding features are that when taken together enable us to reconsider the criteria by which we judge his psychopathology and madness as well as its possible relation to individuation.

Literal Mindedness

As I have referred to it in several places, only a short amplification will be required in order to bring this key feature of Gordon's views on everything into analytical context. The apparent absence of fantasy made him divide his cosmos into a white and black world. The absence of shades and colors of meaning made Gordon an uncompromising, difficult person. Not that he was unable to revert his decisions; quite the contrary, he would, for instance, hand in his resignation one day and take it back the next. But for the moment, each impulsive decision was final. There are several analytical ways of looking at the absence of nuances in the white-and-black world of a literal-minded person like Gordon. We know about Jung's transcendent function which negotiates between real and imaginary data, "thus bridging the yawning gulf between conscious and unconscious" (Jung, 1943 par. 121). But that function does not seem to be working. The same would apply when a person regresses to the paranoid-schizoid position of Melanie Klein. There are further Winnicott's "transitional phenomena," which is a related concept although based on observations of child development. In "Reflections on Not Being Able to Imagine," I mentioned briefly that the imagination of psychotic or borderline patients was limited on account of their hardly being able to distinguish between what was inside or outside themselves, nor between reality and fantasy (Plaut 1966). In his *Transformations*, Bion notes that psychotic patients are unable to think or imagine a situation but have to wait for the thing to appear in external reality (Bion 1965, p. 40). Not surprisingly, there is no symbolic appreciation in these circumstances. I think something of the kind was at work in Gordon. There could be no clearer example than his reference to the communion as the antidote to having eaten the poison of the forbidden fruit. Gordon's statement "a child can understand," i.e., the idea of an antidote, indicates that literal plus magical thinking is operative, rather than symbolic appreciation.

The fundamentalist view of the Bible fitted in well with "a child's understanding." If this mode of thinking appears atavistic to us, we have to remind ourselves that symbolic thinking is a relatively recent acquisition in our evolution. It is a feebly established function and therefore the first to disappear when, not at our best, we regress to the alternative, a mixture of literal and magical thinking. In Gordon's case, this led to a permanent confusion, particularly in areas where for different reasons the senses could not be used to verify his intuitions. This applied particularly to sex and religion. When Gordon nevertheless tried to counteract his confusion by reasoning, as he did in his essay on Eden, a fantastic concoction resulted. It shows how an otherwise sane person can contain psychotic areas where imagination is not available as a bridge between the physical and the symbolical mode of appreciation. Unbridled fantasy then floods the area and confuses both. Here I distinguish, as I did in the paper referred to, between imagination as a form of thinking that can be harnessed to enhance reality and fantasy that cannot. When Gordon was working as an engineer, he could use his imagination and was inventive. But when it came to sexuality, he not only controlled but very nearly stifled his fantasies, presumably because he intuited that they might lead to actions which would bring shame and dishonor upon his head. Homosexual seduction of minors could easily have been his greatest fear. Yet, for his creative imagination, there were outlets that were safe enough. Among these was his ingenuity as a military leader, at which he proved to be outstanding when he had been in command of the Chinese army. Second, there was mapping and sketching. He also had artistic talent as a draftsman. But this, too, had to be tethered to mapping and realistic drawings from nature or photographs.

What I have called literal mindedness and the inability to imagine and to appreciate symbols has an obvious bearing on object relationships, as a passage in the text clearly shows. There he seems to regard it as something of a miracle that ordinary things can become holy in the hands of God and then revert to ordinary again. Instead of seeing these changes as symbolic transformations, they look to Gordon like the transmutation of metals as a realistic possibility might have looked to some alchemists.

Religion

"I hope my dear father and mother think of eternal things . . . Dearest Augusta, pray for me, I beg you." These words were written to his sister, four years older than himself and from an early age Gordon's lifelong confidante, especially in religious matters. Gordon was stationed at the time at Pembroke. He was about age 20 and spent much time in the company of Captain Drew, whose evangelical outlook influenced Gordon. He published religious pamphlets which enabled him to approach strangers and enquire after the state of their souls. One wonders, however, whether he had committed any "sin" for which he asked Augusta to intercede on his behalf, or whether he just regarded her as a pure enough spinster who loved him and could therefore be expected to drop a good word for her brother into God's ear. Anyway, Gordon found a special friend in the divinity and person of Jesus. There can be no doubt that Jesus sacrificing himself *and* wanting to be incorporated by being eaten became the prototype of Gordon's own aspirations. Jesus had become the constant but idealized object that he worshipped and tried to follow. This was the one authority to which Gordon was ready to submit. No doubt, too, that Gordon's interpretation of the crucifixion suited his own death-wish to which I referred earlier ("Who Was Gordon?"). To be dead meant not only to be free from further temptations of the flesh once the soul was freed from the body and rejoined its maker, it also meant a state in which a person "knew all things," thus having become omniscient like the deity itself. As one reads his journals, one becomes aware that Gordon positively envied the dead. As analysts, we have to ask whether, with all his widely acknowledged humility, Gordon projected omniscience and omnipotence onto the deity and hoped for the moment when he could become identical with it, just as God the Father and the Son had become reunited. However this may be, his special relation to Jesus and his attitude toward death cannot be looked at separately. On the phenomenal level, the wish to be dead showed itself, in my view, as fearlessness which impressed everybody who knew him. It may have shown itself already, at the age of nine, while he was staying with his family at Corfu. Although unable to swim, he jumped into deep water and then "waited patiently to be rescued" (MacGregor-Hastie 1985, p. 13). It is also testified for in that he personally led all critical assaults "unarmed, except for a light cane and smoking a cigar," as one news-paper reported. While Governor of the Sudan, he once rode on a camel, again unarmed, into the enemy's camp. Thinking that only a madman or a saint would do such a thing, they must have decided that he was the latter. Anyway, the chief's son, who was in command, kissed his foot and surrender followed. On another occasion, while engaged in the suppressing of the slave trade, he said that he would stop the raids, even if it cost him his life. Everyone knew that he meant it. Finally there was Khartoum, which Gordon had been ordered to evacuate but did not. One biographer, MacGregor-Hastie, asks the pertinent question of whether Gordon really wanted to be rescued and adds, "Is it not possible that he wanted to die, as he did, in a sort of Holy War?" (MacGregor-Hastie 1985, p. 182).

Whatever the connection with his death wish, Gordon's fearless-ness was an inspiration to those who served under him. Whatever the analytic interpretation of his fearlessness, I think that, being the person he was, it took more courage for Gordon to live than to die.

Other features of Gordon's "religion" must be mentioned. One that bears repeating was the love and personal attention he gave to the underprivileged, the sick, and the poor. Did he see his own emotional and sexual deprivation in their plight? Quite likely. Another was that he interspersed his private letters with "D.V." (*deus volens*, God will-ing). Although this was not uncommon in his day, Gordon seems to have sprinkled the D.V. about rather excessively. It was no empty phrase nor just meant as a propitiation of the deity but also, I think, as an expression of his wish truly to submit himself.

Submission seems a strange word to use in connection with Gor-don, whose rebelliousness was widely known and disliked. It had clearly shown itself when he was an officer-cadet and perhaps earlier than that in the form of "mischievousness." As an analyst, one cannot help asking about a man who was in constant trouble with authority what his relationship to his father had been. We have no direct evidence but a number of clues which, when put together, give us intimations. What are they?

1. His father recalled that he did not bawl after birth, but fixed him with bright eyes which had an almost adult expression (MacGregor-Hastie 1985). We don't know what it means, except that his father, a solid establishment figure, had noticed it as peculiar.
2. We recall that Gordon's near insubordinations were the direct

cause of him not entering his father's regiment. Also, he made his reputation serving foreign governments, thus becoming "a soldier of fortune," a title which his father would have particularly disliked (ibid.).

3. Gordon never joined a church, although religious matters were a major preoccupation. He corresponded with clergymen to draw on their knowledge, but in other ways preferred a direct relationship with God. Did he avoid the intermediary of clerical authority? It seems in character.

4. Romolo Gessi, Gordon's close friend for more than twenty-five years was an extroverted Italian who, according to Gordon, knew him so well that it sometimes frightened him (see also Gessi's comments on the *coco de mer* above).

    Why should Gordon have had a foreigner as his friend, someone who was not only different from himself but also from his father? H. W. Gordon had disliked foreigners and was highly esteemed at the War Office, an establishment figure. One may ask whether our Gordon secretly longed for an intimate relationship with his father, as free from all ambivalence as his relationship with God, who was his constantly good and male object. His brothers apparently had no difficulty in conforming and following in their earthly father's footsteps.

5. Analytical curiosity is aroused by his father's death closely coinciding with Gordon's illness which, as he wrote, brought him back to his Saviour. Did he, instead of mourning, project what he may have secretly admired about his father into the heavenly Father?

Although each of these clues may seem highly speculative, when taken together with Gordon's marked and continuous problem with authority, they present presumptive evidence in favor of Gordon's compulsive search for the constantly good father in heaven. It was a search that contributed not a little to him dying the way he did.

Sexuality

Although I have already referred to it in several contexts, the absence of overtly sexual behaviour remains something that arouses curiosity and speculation. Gordon's case demonstrates very clearly that, analytically speaking, it is much more enlightening to consider a person's sexuality in the context of all other traits than to see in it the cause and origin of all troubles. When these are taken together, the whole picture of a person begins to emerge. In our case this means that we have to consider Gordon in relation to his appetites on the one hand and to the search for the constant good object on the other. Both must be looked at against the background of his permanent handicap, his literal mindedness.

The appetite that needs to be given priority, because it must have been the first in his life, is his orality. We remember the wild fantasy about four dozen oysters and the periodic withdrawals accompanied by "B. & S.," Gordon's abbreviation for brandy and soda. Next we have to ask why the paradisiacal apple did not simply cease to exist after it had served Satan as the instrument of temptation. Apparently it became transmuted into the *coco de mer*, alias Eve's pudenda, alias evil. We must conclude that the quality of Satan's instruments remained constant—that is, permanently evil—by contrast with God whose objects, as we saw, went through cyclical changes from ordinary to holy and back. As Gordon had no capacity to appreciate events as symbolic, God's ability to change or, at any rate, temporarily neutralize the poison that had been introduced by oral seduction could only be called miraculous. Gordon does not use the word, but it becomes evident that this is what his "by means," the instrumentality as I called it, signifies. "Miracle" would have brought Gordon too close to Rome. By "unknown means" would have meant a contradiction in terms, an intolerable paradox to the literal mind. Satan's evil ways were by contrast explicable. Like human nature itself, Satan was also irredeemably sinful. Evil could not change as long as the soul remained in the body, that is, during one's lifetime. Satan could use tricks, of course, and change appearances; the unchanging quality of the poison in the paradisiacal apple might *seem* harmless enough but would be revealed by one look at the *coco de mer*. That was no miracle, merely deception. But the Evil One could not trick Gordon, who kept his appetites under strict control. We have seen that this applied to oral and genital appetites. His refusal to take money had also shown itself early on. Analytically this is interpreted as an anal inhibition.

What might have happened, had he allowed himself fantasies in the realm of instinctual drives, does not bear imagining. The Gordon we know could not have lived with himself for an instant.

Conclusion

With this account of Gordon's constant object, psychopathology, and madness in mind, we are now better equipped to return to the criteria by which we judge whether individuation was proceeding.

There can be no doubt about Gordon's constant devotion to the object that could not fail. His faith in it held him together despite all the splitting that made this world black and the world to come white. By being true to the object, Gordon was true to himself as an individual. But was this individuation? Although the theoretical precondition of object constancy remained unfulfilled, I think it was by suffering his psychopathology that the sufferer became more and more himself, unique and different from his fellows whose sympathy he nevertheless aroused. Nor were there any signs of him having become either narcissistically inflated or unduly depressed in the wake of the process, the twin dangers to which Jung had drawn attention. On the other hand, Gordon did not "change" or become different in any way other than becoming more and more himself. It is a moot point whether or not we allow this to be one of the ways in which an individual may change. It is a change in the direction of the "perfection" that, according to Jung, has to be sacrificed. What about completeness? Gordon managed to contain his psychotic area. He did not let his constant object become a preoccupation which would have interfered with his duties and even less a monomanic obsession which would have incurred the label of "psychotic." I suggest that such containment is equivalent to "completeness." Although it is not in line with the analyst's therapeutic aim, this way of self-realization and, as I hold, individuation *is a common phenomenon* in or out of analysis. But in Gordon's case, the self-realization resulted in the fulfillment of the death wish. Whether we regard this as the absolute criterion of a failed individuation is a question beyond the realm of psychology and again involves social and cultural factors.

Putting it like that means challenging the analyst's shibboleth, namely that the patient should change in the course of, or better still, as the demonstrable result of analysis. What is more, the change should be in keeping with his professional ethic, which is not usually questioned when it is in keeping with the prevailing medical and social code. The patient may even be said to have "completely changed." The emphasis is meant as a compliment to the analyst's prowess and must not be taken literally, because that would mean changed beyond recognition and nobody wants to become unrecognizable. On the other hand, we usually mean it as a favorable reaction when we can say of persons that they are "just like themselves." This often means like their lovable, infuriating, or even hateful selves. In any case, the statement indicates that we are pleased to know where we are with someone. Conversely, the reactions of the person so accepted may be agreeable, or they may feel themselves underestimated, even wronged, but still included and recognized as being part of the human race. By contrast, the person who has undergone a "complete change" may well be admired but not necessarily loved, even made to feel like a stranger, left out in the cold. In the case of Gordon, the reactions were mostly of the former kind; wherever he went there was sure to be trouble, but he won admiration as well.

Let us return to the assumption that a person should have coped with his ordinary psychopathology, the gross symptoms or little madnesses, before the process of individuation could begin. Then, in the second stage, so to speak, the person becomes exposed to the twin dangers specific to individuation, namely narcissistic inflation or, alternatively, depression. In Gordon's case there was so much of the ordinary kind that the specific sort remains almost unnoticed, perhaps even doubtful. What there was of inflation in the form of omniscience and omnipotence was projected onto the good and constant object, the deity. With his periodic bouts of depression he was, like everybody else, alone. His Bible was then his only companion and what solace he permitted himself was of the "spiritual kind," in both senses of the word. It is therefore doubtful whether the distinction I drew on earlier between two kinds of psychopathology can be maintained in Gordon's case. Insofar as the sufferer or patient is concerned, there is in any event only one kind of psychopathology; the theoretical differentiation makes no difference to the pain.

Last, what about the severed head that was displayed and mocked in the Mahdi's camp? It is conceivable that analysts would see in it a symbolic confirmation of the split between the controlling superego and the instinctual drives that was one of our hero's characteristics. But if they did, they would be shutting their eyes to an act of barbarism which was in itself the consequence of blind psychotic literal mindedness. To interpret the decapitation symbolically would, in our cultural era, be the symptom of a split and a psychopathology far more dangerous than Gordon's.

It seems ironical that Gordon's design of a crest for the Seychelles after he had "discovered" Eden could have been a fitting epitaph to his own life (figure 7). It shows a palm tree as a central feature, but we

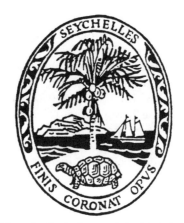

Figure 7. Gordon's crest of the Seychelles.

cannot say whether it is meant to portray one or another of the sacramental trees to which the essay refers. The tortoise is not only a natural inhabitant but is also, according to Jung, primitive and cold-blooded and "symbolizes the instinctual side of the unconscious" (Jung 12, par. 203). The inscription reads "Finis coronat opus," the end crowns the work, and requires no comment.

References

Bion, W. R. 1965. *Transformations*. London: William Heinemann Medical Books, Ltd.

Gordon, C. G. 1882. Eden and its two sacramental trees. Unpublished manuscript.

Gordon, H. W. 1885. *Events in the Life of Charles George Gordon*. London: Kegan Paul.

Hartmann, H. 1964. *Essays on Ego Psychology*. London: Hogarth Press.

Jung, C. G. 1931. The stages of life. In *CW* 8:387–403. Princeton, N.J.: Princeton University Press, 1969.

———. 1943. On the psychology of the unconscious. In *CW* 7:3–121. Princeton, N.J.: Princeton University Press, 1953.

———. 1944. *Psychology and Alchemy. CW* vol. 12. Princeton, N.J.: Princeton University Press, 1953.

MacGregor-Hastie, R. 1985. *Never to Be Taken Alive*. London: Sedwick and Jackson.

Milton, J. 1666. Paradise Lost. *Milton's Poetical Works*, Douglas Bush, ed. Oxford: University Press, 1979.

Nutting, A. 1966. *Gordon: Martyr and Misfit*. London: Constable.

Plaut, A. 1966. Reflections on not being able to imagine. *Journal of Analytical Psychology* 11,2:121.

———. 1974. Part-object relations and Jung's "Luminosities." *JAP* 19,2:175.

———. 1982. General Gordon's map of paradise. *Encounter* (June/July) 58/59, 6/1:20–32.

_____. 1991. Object constancy or constant object. In *Psychopathology, Contemporary Jungian Perspectives*, A. Samuels, ed. London: Karnac Books.

Rycroft, C. 1968. *A Critical Dictionary of Psychoanalysis*. London: Nelson.

Strachey, L. 1918. *Eminent Victorians*. Harmondsworth: Penguin Modern Classics, 1980.

Trench, C. C. 1978. *Charley Gordon: An Eminent Victorian Reassessed*. London: Alan Lane.

A Response to "General Gordon's Constant Object" by Fred Plaut

Ronald B. Kledzik

Reading Dr. Plaut's paper brought back memories of the first time I heard of him. It was back in the early sixties just after I had arrived in Zürich to begin training. Jung had been dead only a few months, and the second or third International Jungian Congress was to begin just a few days after I got there. I still recall the enormous tension in the air at that Congress, which centered around the question of Kleinian theory and its importance in Jungian psychology.

At the time I didn't know what a Kleinian was; but whatever the crisis was about, the fires were really turned up, and it was obvious that neither side would give an inch to the other.

Now you must realize that this was some time ago, during the very last days of the heroic period of Jungian psychology. Or, to put it another way, no matter where you turned in that Congress, you were already knee-deep in activated primitive object relations.

It happened that just before the Congress I had picked up the first Jungian journal I had ever seen and read an article by one Alfred Plaut. I've forgotten the subject of the article but never the author. This Dr. Plaut wrote with absolute fierceness. As I recall, he was defending some

Ronald B. Kledzik is assistant professor of psychiatry and a Jungian analyst in private practice in Virginia Beach, Virginia. A graduate of the C. G. Jung Institute in Zürich, he is interested in cultural psychology, borderline conditions and narcissism, and art therapy.

argument, and he literally leveled the field around him for miles in every direction. So when I got to the Congress and saw Dr. Plaut's name on the program, I thought, "This is going to be a free-for-all," and indeed it was a humdinger of a Congress with, as I remember, one group of Jungians getting up and walking out to join the Kleinians. But Dr. Plaut! He never even drew his sword. Instead he spoke quietly and reflectively, refusing to be drawn into battle. That was my first — and lasting — impression of you, Fred.

Dr. Plaut comments at the beginning of his paper that instead of a clinical case, he has presented a historical figure removed from us by a century and a half. In doing so, he has given us an added possibility of viewing General Gordon within the historical context of prepsychological, nineteenth-century Victorian England, and I hope that at some point Dr. Plaut will say more about the cultural influences on General Gordon's life.

But over and above this, the goal of Dr. Plaut's paper is to present a concept of his own, namely that of the constant object as well as its relationship to psychopathology, madness, and the individuation process, and he does this by using a study of General Charlie Gordon, a nineteenth-century English army officer of considerable fame.

Dr. Plaut describes the concept of the constant object largely in comparison to object constancy, i.e., whole object relatedness which, in such borderline individuals as General Gordon, has not been achieved. Using the language of Melanie Klein, Dr. Plaut defines his concept simply as the good constant object. We will come back to this later.

I would like to start at the end of Dr. Plaut's paper where he considers the individuation process from the constant object point of view. There he takes pains to explain that, in terms of individuation, the constant object is no mere substitute, no pale imitation, as it were, of object constancy, but instead a vital alternative which can be therapeutic, growth producing, and, as, Dr. Plaut strongly implies, ultimately a way of individuation. I say "implies" rather than "is" a way of individuation because, although I believe the latter is Dr. Plaut's position, I couldn't find such a declarative statement in his paper. Perhaps he would state this more definitely or elaborate upon why he might hesitate to do so.

Concerning the constant object itself, Dr. Plaut wrote a paper on this concept in 1975, which ideally we should have as a companion paper to his present one, for in it are several ideas which belong organically to his paper today. I'll mention two of them which bring together concepts from object relations theory and analytical psychology theory where the two meet and overlap. In comparing object constancy with the constant object, he wrote that the latter can be classified neither as good nor bad in the Kleinian sense, but, instead, it is fascinating, awe-inspiring, in short, numinous. Now this is somewhat daring, because Jung never said it; and to many, what Jung has not said may not be worth saying. Then at the very end of that paper Dr. Plaut takes a giant step by suggesting that the constant object may indeed be identical with Jung's concept of the Self, and while he uses a somewhat specula-tive tone for the latter idea, it is nevertheless in line with the assertion in the present paper that God or the Deity was General Gordon's constant object. So, in a spirit of synthesis, Dr. Plaut is saying that his concept of the constant object and Jung's idea of the Self partake of sameness, which immediately brings up the question of the presence of the opposites of good and evil within the Jungian Self, and the absence of good and bad in Plaut's constant object. Perhaps this is an abstruse question, but could the Kleinian good and bad be absent within the constant object while the Jungian notion of good and evil remains? Otherwise, viewing the self (or God) as containing both good and evil would, theoretically anyway, appear to disqualify its serving as the all-good constant object. Having spoken with Dr. Plaut about this ques-tion, I know that his response will open the door to several interesting and relevant ideas.

Dr. Plaut speaks of numinosity as being a characteristic of the constant object, implying that if one acquires a constant object, it is via a numinous experience. We know of the importance Jung gave to the numinosum as the healing factor par excellence. So what about the people who have achieved object constancy? What is their path to the numinous? For example, take the biblical Saul on the road to Damas-cus. Let us assume that he was a good Roman citizen, well integrated into the establishment and possessed of most of the trappings of object constancy. Then came the numinous experience. How could he remain in object constancy after that? Did Saul perhaps have to sacrifice object constancy in order to become Paul? Taking this clinically, must a patient sacrifice object constancy, if he or she possesses it, to approach the numinous? Also, in terms of the experience (numinous) of acquir-ing the constant object, do mad parts come as part of the deal, so to speak, or does the constant object offer a way to deal with already present mad parts?

Until now I thought I understood object constancy, but I really don't. I found myself thinking that a person with solid object constancy wouldn't have mad parts, or conversely, that the ego in failing to achieve object constancy creates mad parts. Clearly inferior thinking, but it points up the need, Dr. Plaut, for you to say a little bit about how some people seem to end up with mad parts and others don't.

Now, staying just a moment longer in Kleinian territory, let us consider General Gordon's constant object in terms of the Kleinian concept of the good breast. You recall Gordon's famous map which, after he had definitely located Paradise upon it, became the preoccupation of his life. Well, it turns out that Christopher Columbus thought similarly but in more graphic terms. Columbus wrote that in sailing the unknown waters to the West Indies, he fully expected to pass by the original site of the biblical Paradise.

It would be recognizable, he said, because Paradise would be on that part of the earth closest to heaven, which he explained by saying that the earth was not exactly round but shaped more like a pear with the protruding narrow end holding Paradise on its tip. Now it may well be an eccentricity of cartographers and world travelers to see the world this way, but Columbus fully expected to see Paradise as he sailed up and over the tip of the pear.

I mention this anecdote because it points to the origin in Kleinian theory of Dr. Plaut's concept. I would ask Dr. Plaut to describe the factors involved in the evolution of a simply good object—the good breast—into his constant object.

In your paper, Dr. Plaut, you go to some lengths to show the similarities between the tasks of object constancy and those of the constant object, namely, that both require successfully facing the twin dangers of depression and narcissistic inflation, both require suffering one's psychopathology, both involve achieving at least some degree of completeness or self-realization, etc. Nevertheless, your emphasis is upon the "otherness" of the constant object path, namely, that it offers the ego an opportunity to consolidate around a different center, to integrate around a different core than that provided by object constancy. My question: Does the difference between these two paths lead to different kinds of self-structure, specifically, does it create two typologically different personalities?

A further question along this line, more general in nature: If we exclude organized religions, where do people who take the path of the constant object today tend to gravitate in society? Have you seen many in therapy?

And, one last question in this regard, and, Fred, this one doesn't have to be answered. Considering both of the above kinds of people, do you think that the object constancy group has established at least a foothold in the Jungian community?

Which brings me to my last consideration: General Gordon and his madness. But first, I take my hat off to the General because he accomplished what he did with the benefit of neither the church nor an analyst. He had nothing on his side except personal faith in his good constant object.

I would like to look briefly at his life in its cultural context, namely Victorian England. If, as Dr. Plaut has mentioned, nineteenth-century England was at the height of the Empire, so was it also under the power of the titanic Victorian Ego, an awesome psychological construct, the downside of which not only explicitly suppressed sexuality and sexual imagination, but stifled personal fantasy of all kinds as well. Respectability and honor were raised to cult status, which demanded standards of self-discipline that have been described as simply inhuman.

General Gordon, then, was the consummate Victorian: an exemplary soldier, self-sacrificing and fearless, possessed of a will of steel, a man who avoided any known sexuality, and who was, by our standards anyway, severely limited in his ability to fantasize. It is upon this latter characteristic of General Gordon's that I wish to focus: his literal mindedness. Dr. Plaut writes that the imagination of psychotic or borderline individuals is limited on account of their hardly being able to distinguish between what is inside or outside themselves, nor between reality and fantasy.

He goes on to add an observation of Bion's that psychotic patients are unable to imagine a situation but instead must wait for it to appear in external reality, i.e., literally.

In General Gordon's case, it seems that when he was abroad, on the road as a soldier, what he could not imagine met him in the form of madness. For example, to walk unarmed and alone into the headquarters of the enemy camp may be brilliant, but it is insane; leading his troops into battle with only a light cane and smoking a cigar may inspire his soldiers, but it is insane; and refusing instructions to evacuate Khartoum is stupid as well as insane.

So it seems likely that General Gordon's dramatic military exploits abroad served as the place in external reality where he met, as it were, in the Chinese and Africans, his own—and his culture's—split-off internal parts, against which he quite psychotically warred and finally martyred himself.

Strangely, as Dr. Plaut points out, General Gordon volunteered himself for these military ventures, which, it seems to me, took him away from the constant good object and off his path of individuation. Perhaps simply he could not outlast his psychopathology and chose instead to identify with his good object Jesus and die as a martyr.

War, Madness, and the Morrigan, a Celtic Goddess of Life and Death

Sylvia Brinton Perera

A political situation is the manifestation of a parallel psychological problem in millions of individuals. This problem is largely unconscious (which makes it a particularly dangerous one!).

Jung, *Letters I: 1906–1950,* p. 535

The war in the Persian Gulf had an intense impact on many Americans even though most of us do not live in close geographic proximity to the palpable atrocities of war. We were not under bombardment. Nor did we have to flee our homes and endure thirst, starvation, and exposure. We did not have to don gas masks while

---

This paper is part of a work in progress on Celtic mythological themes. It has been adapted from a presentation to the C. G. Jung Society of New Mexico on May 25, 1991. I want here to express my thanks for the stimulating discussion with members of the Society and with colleagues at The Woman's Gathering, an annual women's retreat that developed out of the Chiron conferences. I am especially grateful to Karin Carrington, Morgan Farley, Robbie Goodman, Celeste Miller, and Carol Zeitz for their comments. I also wish particularly to thank Suzi Naiburg for her editorial help and E. Christopher Whitmont for his encouragement in the course of writing my way through this material.

Sylvia Brinton Perera is a member of the New York Association of Analytical Psychology, a teacher at the C. G. Jung Institute of New York, and a practicing analyst in New York and Connecticut. She is the author of *Descent to the Goddess: A Way of Initiation for Women, The Scapegoat Complex: Toward a Mythology of Shadow and Guilt,* and co-author of *Dreams, A Portal to the Source.*

living under the threat of chemical attack. We were fortunate. Nonetheless, many of us deeply felt the collective tensions of the war's buildup after Iraq invaded Kuwait in August 1990.[1] In January and February 1991, we participated on a more personal level via concerned connection to individuals living or serving in the Middle East, our fear of terrorism, and television images of the war itself. Many of us are still participating emotionally in the upheaving horrors of the war's aftermath. The Gulf War brought vast human destruction and environmental pollution. It also precipitated increased consciousness of global issues and the Gulf area's problems. For some of us, the images of war facilitated the uncovering of psychotic pockets in ourselves as functioning adults, permitting old wounds to open and, in some cases, healing initiations to begin.

Several psychoanalysts told me they had never had to contain and metabolize so much primal emotion in analysands at once, never saw so many urban and suburban middle-class clients catapulted at one time into fear, despair, and emotional chaos. Those of us concerned with global and personal ecology know these emotions are relatively common in an age of catastrophic upheavals and in the process of analytic work. What marked this period as different was the acute nature of the effects of what the military called a "desert storm" on both neurotic analysands and on those functioning at more infantile or borderline levels. Its effects were similar to those of a sudden natural disaster or family death, because the war opened the psyche to anguish, fear of annihilation, impotence, rage, chaotic fragmentation, and loss of meaning. It gave many otherwise insulated people a taste of what many third world and ghetto populations live with on a daily basis.

The psychotherapeutic literature was full of articles about the war's impact on daily life. "A constant barrage of television, newspaper, and magazine coverage has brought the Persian Gulf war into almost every American's living room," wrote *The Psychiatric Times* in March 1991. "The electronic media is covering new ground with regard to the vividness and immediacy of war images, and no viewer is able to remain remote—cognitively or affectively—from these stimuli" (Wagner 1991). "Counselors in all sorts of settings report that their clients are having anxiety attacks, increased anger reactions, reduced frustration tolerance and other similar symptoms that can be traced directly or indirectly to Desert Storm" (Hacker 1991a). "Post traumatic stress reactions may now surface . . . [among] returning military personnel, but in other clients as well . . . Adults and children in the general population may need counseling, especially those who have gone through trauma or crisis, as they see pictures of the war and its victims" (Hacker, 1991b).

Part of the initial potency of the war in our psyches was due to the continuous television barrage of immediate war pictures, what was commonly referred to in New York as "CNN fever." As Jungians we know that images can compel consciousness and libido. Our psyches are always using and reacting to images of outer phenomena. Everything from day residues to large, collective events and natural catastrophes may interface with our inner processes. The Gulf War provided a prime manifestation of the vital and perhaps ultimately world-saving fact that we live in a new age, one in which telecommunications enable us to experience far events as near, hidden events as exposed, even ones we would like to deny as real. The shadow side of this awareness is a capacity in television viewers to become excessively preoccupied with repetitions of scenes that arouse anxiety and cause them to defend against their fear by denying or trivializing what they see. In our attacks of CNN fever, we were gripped by video images. Our empathy and horror were deeply stirred. As the war progressed, the news became more carefully guarded. Even as we rationally understood the military necessity for censorship, we hungered more anxiously for accurate information. Frustrated, we focused on the television source as if it were a seductive, persecutory, and withholding mother. Eager to take in whatever we saw, we were then forced to swallow the same exciting and disturbing images over and over again, because nothing fresh was forthcoming fast enough.

Bombarded by media coverage and empathically joined to family members and neighbors stationed across the globe, we were ineluctably drawn to share imaginally and emotionally in distant events and to recognize our interconnectedness with those in a remote and yet utterly immediate and palpable world. Most of us were privileged and blessed to be only participant observers of catastrophe. Our survival was not dependent upon taking such necessary actions as seeking refuge in bomb shelters or sealing off rooms against the threat of chemical attack. Actions of all kinds — those required for safety and survival and those we chose to do thousands of miles away from the war theater — helped to mute raw emotional responses. One friend in Haifa told me she felt her terror focused on her children under bombardment in Tel Aviv, because she was not near them and felt helpless to protect them. Nonetheless, necessary acts such as securing tape around the openings of the community's bomb shelter distracted and calmed her. Simple routines like the nightly ritual of gathering what would be needed when the air-raid warnings sounded functioned as guardians and made sleep possible.[2] A Muslim friend in New York began to organize relief work. Her action, too, was an outlet for unbearable emotion and helped her to feel more closely connected to those who were endangered. In the United States, many people roused themselves to act and counsel families with spouses or parents in the Gulf, march in demonstrations, write letters to service people, and even display yellow ribbons. Such actions help to channel and mitigate whole-body responses.[3] Other actions — such as attending prayer vigils or participating in discussion groups — met needs for containment and community. Such transmutations of anxiety into assertive action and dependent bonding have been found to be characteristic of neurotics under threat of war (Ierodiakonou 1970, pp. 643 ff).

Far from actual disaster, many of us nevertheless felt the potency of multiple, repeated, and intense images of war. They broke through the electronic buffer zone we like to think television offers. Many of us sat at home feeling ourselves assaulted by media images, which fell like bombs into our psyches gashing open deeply buried emotions. Because the immediacy of the television images hit us vividly and repeatedly with a power that destroyed normal boundaries between outer and inner, collective and personal, present and past, we were often forced into depth where our own oldest wounds are scarred over. This may have been particularly true of those engaged in deep analytic work either as analysands or analysts. One analysand who viewed the early scenes of war said: "I am compelled — that's the word — to watch the news. Some awful truth out there has stretched open a tunnel to anarchy that I already know and don't want to know — an inside battlefield bombardment that feels close to the outer madness. . . ." Another analysand afflicted by the archaic level unleashed somatically and emotionally in his psyche by the barraging images of Desert Storm complained, "I closed that stuff, but this war is opening up an old wound, and I have to be a hero and go back and look at intolerable pains in me as much as I have to look at the news, [because] . . . my old, buried, inner pain merges with the present fear and chaos. It gets pulled into the light as if by a magnet. . . . But I feel as helpless now as ever I did then."

The media and military attempted to erect primitive defenses of depersonalization and dissociation as they sought to make us feel we were watching a video game rather than people like ourselves under those elegantly precise, computerized cruciform bomb sites. How often we heard not about the human deaths but only about "collateral damage." The military and the media spoke of a "turkey shoot" on the road to Basra when the fleeing armies were so easily killed. Many people were deeply disturbed by the crazy communication patterns and weird reversals of some of the feeding media, which spoke of devastating bombing raids as if they were sport, of war actions as a video game, of missiles as "smart,"[4] and of fireworks at a baseball game weeks after the hostilities had ended as missiles in the skies over Baghdad (*New York Times*, April 21, 1991). Such dissociation and reversals replicate magic-level and psychotic communications, which create perceptual and cognitive dissonances that were often close to schizophrenogenic. The metaphors forced a painful jarring of cognitive categories and were often felt as sadistic. One woman was reminded of her father's habit of venting his sadism by throwing his keys at his children's elbows when they rested them on the dining table while he blithely proved that he had not lost his baseball pitcher's aim.

An analysand who is also a therapist wrote about the onslaught of chaotic devastation in her own psyche that she experienced on the night of January 16, 1991, when she had inadvertently turned on the news:

> Bombs are falling in Baghdad. The ancient city of empires that once conjured up magic lanterns, jewel-colored carpets, and the attar of roses and oil is tonight devastated by modern weapons and tyranny and war. Tonight as the people slept, I have seen their city stalked from the air and suddenly prey to deadly explosives. I have seen it ringed in the light of tracer bullets and bombs. Sitting here, waiting for friends for dinner in New York, I have seen war falling from the skies onto Baghdad as if I were inside the distant city, sharing the horror of the people there. Weirdly we here could know what our forces are doing to them before our own commanders announced it and before they even knew its effects.

> I feel shaken in my core. Some always-assumed order has collapsed before my eyes and ears. The endangered TV crew presented the truth raw to my/our senses. No safely distancing authority censored or told us what to believe. That feels as momentous an overturning of the hierarchy of safety as reading the vernacular Bible must have felt to medieval Catholic minds.

> I feel shattered. All rational boundaries tumble into an abyss. Time is collapsing. Effect seemed to come before cause. Space collapses. I see from within ravaged Baghdad, which I view from inside my safe Manhattan room, the immediate, cataclysmic results there/here of the enemy's enemy—ourselves. I feel fear, excitement, horror, despair, fascination, helplessness. Especially helplessness. I did not want this; I have worked all fall to avoid it, but I am now deeply part of it. Yet I am still here; safe and helpless and suffering helplessness and fear like some catastrophe inside me.

> Where is this going, this rough beast unleashed and horribly slouching so near to Bethlehem? I would like to pray but I have only chaotic fear and confusion to be a prayer. Evil is on all sides, and sudden awesome destruction. I can only

stare into the chaos that is over us all. Cruelty and disorder beyond justice,
beyond mind.

The chaotic war images triggered catastrophic psychological upheavals
in certain sensitive individuals. In such times of crisis when we cannot
maintain our habitual psychological defenses and patterns of coping,
we may suffer profound confusion and are thereby propelled into real-
izations that may otherwise have been much slower in forming. Such a
transformation in order to form a new consciousness or achieve a new
integration does not seem to develop without each of us going through
a period of what the alchemists called dismemberment and *nigredo*.
Periods of emotional turbulence and chaos may actually prepare the
way for transformation. The Gulf War gave those of us who were
intensely involved as participant observers an opportunity for a short,
potent, and blessedly safe-enough descent into chaos that overwhelms
or dismembers the ego. We know that such descents can take us into
borderline and psychotic layers in the psyche where our own pockets of
still-unworked complexes make us susceptible to dismemberment. We
know that such descents may be transformative if we can work through
our personal complexes and find meaningful images around which
create a new integration. As one analysand poignantly said: "The
images and emotions out there pierce through me. I feel torn apart
because I feel both sides are wrong. I can't flee to any fragment of this
mess to hold me because there is nothing to polarize my fear against
. . . to make a hated adversary and make me a whole against it . . . I
know I need to seek a higher integration, but where is an image to
integrate this chaos?"

The Mother of All Battles

Most often we think of war as conflict between opposing parties,
and our concern is with power, right and wrong, winning and losing,
and/or conflict resolution. We coalesce ourselves, as this analysand
could not do, by pitting ourselves aggressively against an adversary. A
group or nation, too, can pull itself together by facing a common
enemy. By focusing attention on external threat, we may divert ourselves from domestic issues. We may also distance ourselves from the
emotional impact of war by assessing combat skills, strategy, and weap-
onry. After the war is over, we may try to explore the historical, economic, cultural, and inevitable archetypal roots of such profoundly
acted-out discord. We talk in abstractions about attachment and hostil-
ity, love and death instincts, or in terms of biological drives or testoster-

one levels. We differentiate aggression into the libido that fuels interspecies mating fights and that which forces combat against outsiders. We look at power, at issues of domination, and the need for outlets for power and aggression. We talk about nations playing robber and policeman/messiah and about the inflations that are inevitable as both sides proclaim that God is theirs alone. We try to manage the archetypal potency of war with rituals, war games, and strategies of conflict resolution (Stevens 1989; Bernstein 1989, pp. 79–124).

As Jungians we speak of war—whether enacted or experienced between nations or experienced in the individual psyche—as a conflict between opposites. On the psychological level, we are trained to use the imaginal realm and the transcendent function to find some grace of a reconciling third position. On both psychological and political levels, we look at issues of the shadow and shadow projection onto the enemy. We explore how we distance from and dehumanize the other, transforming the enemy into a nonhuman demon so that we are free to vent our hate and destructiveness without empathy (Keen 1986).

Such shadow levels came up in some clients' material. One man had consciously identified with what we were told was a brainwashed POW and told his therapist, "I [also] learned to say anything to get the brutes off my back." After this was explored with reference to his communications to his therapist, he then dreamed that Saddam Hussein was sitting in his new kitchen waiting for him to come home. The dreamer initially identified the figure of the dictator with his mother, saying it "represents sadism—a torturing power that does not care, that has no bounds to cruelty, destruction, and greed." The therapist also saw the figure as a reference to her previous confrontation, for the dreamer tended to experience such powerful destructiveness in women, and this projection had often made him feel at the mercy of his wife, girlfriends, and therapist. After the transferential implications had been discussed, the dreamer mused on the image of the Iraqi leader. He began to push out his chest. When his attention was drawn to his change in posture, he noticed how it conveyed his pleasure in raw, chthonic, dominative power—a shocking idea to him but one that he had to meet in his own personal kitchen, the psychological place of cooking and transformation. As we worked on the dream image over several weeks, he began to acknowledge his own power shadow and to realize that "such power capable of the worst horrors of war might be part of me."

The deeper existential level that the Gulf War opened in my clients and friends and in myself includes issues of inner conflict and shadow confrontation; however, it has been better named in the hyperbole of the Arabs as "The Mother of All Battles." This phrase is actually an English translation of the Arabic, but it holds an image of the matrix of primary consciousness beneath polarizations and warring conflict. Thus, it does indeed belong to and encompass both sides. This Terrible Mother is an ancient, archetypal image of war, which we know from various mythologies. Once more its archetypal meaning and powerful horror crashed into our contemporary psyches. Public figures acted to mute the dread that the phrase conveyed. It quickly became a catchword in this country after its initial impact subsided and we became confident we would decimate Iraq's forces from the air. With repetition, we drained the phrase of its grim power. We reduced it to a mere slogan that proved our strength against the Terrible Mother of Death. Headlines referred to "The Mother of All Defeats." To dispel lingering terror in New York, Mayor Dinkins began to speak of the ticker-tape homecoming of U.S. troops as "The Mother of All Parades." General Schwarzkopf, who led the allied victory on the field and, in his television interviews, mediated both the hysteria of some newscasters and the chaos of the war itself, was named "Father of the Year." He carried the archetypal role needed to balance the terrible Mother of All Battles.

Nonetheless, the phrase and the images we were compelled to watch on television opened many of us to experiences of the Terrible Mother of Life and Death and the primal, painful, overwhelming affects of her children. For a short time, she possessed us and drove many of us into states we associate with psychosis. One particularly susceptible client expressed this horror when she said she feared the end of the world. She suffered acute diarrhea in her panic throughout the weeks of combat. For her, this war held the terrible danger of apocalypse—of global annihilation, the primeval terror that underlies all our undoing and fuels the fires that overwhelm consciousness and bring on psychosis. Many people were initially scared of the realistic potential of nuclear involvement and the terrifying, boundary-violating chemical and gas weapons. This client's belief that the apocalypse was imminent exacerbated such realistic collective dangers. She felt her sense of ordered limits and security on earth eroded just as profoundly as nameless fears of annihilation undermine the psychotic's ego.

In this war, too, the use of hi-tech equipment gave some of us a strange sense that something awesome and nonhuman was in charge of an unfathomable horror. At the primitive, autistic level of consciousness, there is no experience of safe human boundaries to define and protect the psyche's body ego. Things, parts of things and people, and shapes substitute for human beings and are often felt as invasively threatening. The war's unleashing of awesome inhuman power replicates early experience of parental caretakers as all-powerful impersonal forces in charge of events we had to suffer, and it touches the numinosity of relationships between ego and Self, between human and divine or demonic.

Many people palpably experienced a fear of terrible Fate and an unknowable maw into which they expected that life might plunge. This terror exposed an underlying sense of helplessness and a felt lack of protection from giant, arbitrary forces. While this helpless fear led some people to church to seek spiritual connection, containment, and an outlet for dependency needs, it also led some to deep analytic work. The images and feelings outside provoked by the Gulf War reverberated deeply into old personal experiences of fear and helplessness before sadistic and chaotic caretakers—the terrible parent of all battles and defeats.

Inevitably, those for whom the external collective crisis touched the deepest levels of the psyche were individuals with early personal experiences of terror in the face of helplessness, annihilation, chaos, and erruptive primary emotions. They could identify with the vulnerability and impotence of both soldiers and civilians, because their own histories of childhood abuse or neglect made "the frightening images they see on television . . . resonate with their early perceptions of an unsafe world" (Yudofsky, quoted in Wagner 1991). Some defended against the news by avoiding it altogether because it stirred too painfully into old traumata with which they were not ready to deal. One client, denying any "particular interest" in the war was, however, seized with asthma attacks when the war began. These replicated a long-gone, childhood problem. As we worked on the reactive somatic symptom, he realized that he was terrified that his only son, who had just turned nineteen, might be drafted and killed. Underneath his immediate and realistic concern, he found the old symptom of asthma also pointed his attention to his own childhood terror of annihilation now projected where there was a poignant reality hook to carry the problem.

For many of us, the boundaries between group and individual, outer and inner were stretched thin and often torn. What was manifesting collectively opened resonating wounds in personal psychology, and these reciprocally alerted us to the depth of destruction and madness in war. Conversely, what was an individual and chronic "psychotic pocket" in personal psychology was manifesting collectively, and it was gripping. One man felt compelled to watch the news for hours even though it meant abandoning ongoing personal projects. He said, "My work, my family, life itself feels trivial in the face of the horrors out there." This was a rather common feeling—that daily life palled before such grim intensities. In his case, however, the compulsion to sit by the news and feel anxious had a magic quality: "By watching and feeling so much worry, at least I am doing something. Maybe it even helps." As we worked on his reactions, he discovered memories of his chronically sick mother, whom he began to realize he had also sat beside and watched, hating her absence from his active life and also giving her the gift of all he had then, which was his participant anguish. Defending against unspeakable helplessness, he had used anxiety magically in both the past and present situations.

Some people I know and/or work with had only passing reactions to the war, for their own lives were either in a personal chaos that dwarfed the events across the globe, or they were involved in deeply introverted processes.[5] Some of those least touched by the events of the war were preoccupied with their own creative projects. Two pregnant clients were focused on the life processes within them. One writer forced himself to stay with his novel. Each of these three felt engaged in consciously asserting an alternative to destruction.

One client was overwhelmed with gratitude for a television commentator's concern about children's fear of the war and furious at a reporter who dismissed a child's questions about his own fear to speak only about needing to perform his job well. The dismissal reminded her of how she had experienced her father's abandoning the family in wartime Europe to go off dutifully and "act the hero." She could vent fury at the reporter she had never allowed herself to feel or express against her father, whose leaving was felt to be an emotional rejection. She was, however, fascinated and relieved to follow the reports of officers helping soldiers in the field discuss their fears of mutilation, gassing, and death. "The macho world of denial, even in the army, is shifting. I wish my father had lived to hear that it is all right to have feelings."

With other clients, the war's violence reverberated into their own personal, primal fears of annihilation and brought to consciousness a personal existential anguish and feelings of lack of containment in a terrifyingly vast and dangerous universe. The war reevoked childhood terrors before experiences of boundlessness, chaos, inner and outer explosiveness, and memories of zombielike defenses against overwhelming hate and violence. As one woman said, "If you don't feel safe on earth anyway, then this war makes life nearly impossible." She

experienced the sudden rearousal of her victimized child complex as the
images of bombing replicated fears of her raging alcoholic mother, who
had "invaded—like war from the skies." Lurched into parallel emotional resonance, she also began to reexperience her attempts to "play
dead and numb out" to avoid being the target of her mother's violent
attention.

Another client, normally a competent professional, was so fearful
of terrorism he could not even make the trip to therapy. He was convinced he would be blasted by terrorists in the train station or airport.
The outer reality of such a possibility was felt by several out-of-town
clients, by many New Yorkers in public spaces, by commuters who
bought up all the gas masks available in New York, fearing terrorism in
the train stations, and by those who cancelled air reservations. This
client was plunged unexpectedly into inchoate fear and felt ashamed of
his cowardice, for it belied his persona of competence. Working in
therapy by phone, we explored his terror of terrorism as an objective
reaction to real threat that showed he was guarding himself as no one
had cared for him as a child. Gradually we began to uncover specific
memories under the nameless dread. His maternal uncle and abusive
brother had blasted his body boundaries from outside when he was a
boy, just as his own overwhelming feelings of terror and rage had
blasted his psychic boundaries from inside, because no one had mediated his emotional reactions to the early physical abuse. He began to
remember how it felt to be treated inhumanly and brushed aside as if
he were merely "collateral damage." He realized he never expected to
be treated like a human being. He dreamed of a cockroach that lay in
his bed. In his associations, he recalled a television interview with one
pilot who had helped bomb the Iraqi Republican Guard. "They look,"
the pilot had said, "just like cockroaches." The client readily identified
himself as a lowly but surviving cockroach who had lived in darkness,
hiding all his life behind his persona. Nonetheless, he projected an
explosive terrorism onto strangers lurking in Penn Station. The right-
eous ruthlessness of the Republican Guard sometimes erupted unconsciously through him. His wife complained about sudden outbursts of
panicky rage with which he blasted his family when they disobeyed his
fanatic requirements. The dream and his associations of the cockroach
with the Republican Guard point toward a conscious potential to mediate assertion and guard himself in a way that would make cockroach
hiding unnecessary. While still identified with the fragile victim of
attack, this potential is still in thrall, like the Republican Guard, to an
inner sadistic and tyrannical superego that substitutes for ego strength

and the Self's authority. In the dream, the lowly cockroach is still in bed. But it came out of hiding to be seen as he hid himself away from the "dangerous trip" to therapy.

Fear of gas attacks roused terror in many people whose relatives had died in the Holocaust. The image of Israeli civilians and reporters in their shelters fumbling to put on their masks haunted one client as if it was her own experience of traumatic stress. The image leapt over and over into her mind to reevoke the nameless dread that had hung over her family. She retreated to her bed, the one place of safety she remembered from childhood. Only when she could ground her current sense of fearful helplessness in her own parallel childhood experience did she find some relief. This occurred as she vividly began to remember a series of painful operations she had undergone before she was six, that made her feel mutilated. She spoke of the repeated experiences of anaesthesia:

> I thought I would die each time, like the relatives in the camp showers. And I would wake up hurting, but no one wanted to hear about it. They told me I was lucky, and I held onto that. I made myself believe it finally. I never wanted to look at this again, but that gas mask scene and the terror of chemical weapons are bringing it all back . . . I know that fear. It's an attack on my body, just like on theirs. The dread then was like an evil gas that erodes me, unnames me, so I was less than nothing. [Note how the present and past are fused.] And there was no one to communicate myself with. So I was gone, like the tree in the forest no one hears falling. And I could not speak from within my fear; I was told I was foolish. So I still think I was bad, even evil, for having fear and hurting, when others had had it so much worse . . . It's a relief to talk now, but scary. Then I felt chopped up into pieces that got smaller and smaller. And I died as if there was something wrong with me like the Jews in the showers. Eventually I got myself renamed to myself as this big, coping superwoman, who can't really manage, who can't really feel . . . But this war has undermined me again . . . Imagine, I have collapsed with just one television scene!

Her experience of being "gone like the tree in the forest" had crept like gas through her life to create an underlying dissociated numbness. When she first came into therapy, she was still cutting herself with nails to "feel something" and to fasten herself into reality—albeit a reality of suffering. Now, several years after she had stopped cutting herself, she was still the victim of attacks of hysterical fear that gave her a sense of aliveness and wild energy even as they incapacitated her. The war gave her another opportunity to return to the underlying archaic dread and express more of it in a secure, empathic and contained space.

Almost everyone was appalled by Saddam's environmental

terrorism—the spilling of oil onto the sea and the burning of oil fields. Images of the oil-covered, helpless cormorants (actually taken from another oil spill but epitomizing the current issue) touched us viscerally. As one woman said, "We look at raw evil here, the wanton use of power to destroy nature and innocent creatures that are not even party to this madness. Now I feel hate and rage." Again, the outer collective scene touched an inner personal chord. In the alchemical way that is central to analytic work, this client worked across the thin membrane from collective to personal. She felt an upsurge of identification with the helpless bird, of the helplessness and rage she had experienced as a small child. Exploring what was both a realistic and a complex reaction, she remembered "body memories of abuse to my body—caretakers who did invasive things . . . medical procedures . . . a hospital stay where children screamed and I was as silent as a stunned rabbit, alone in my bed, hiding from awful 'procedures' that were supposed to be good attention. . . . Now," she said,

> I can feel enraged for the cormorants and fish and the people whose waters are spoiled. I want to kick and scream, to kill the abusers. But again I feel so helpless and hopeless. The war machines are rolling. As a child when I was helpless, I learned to get quiet and retreat so far inside I became a tiny, hard ball, and I never really knew what was inside that. Maybe it is the rage I feel now as all those memories of frailty and fear are just like what I feel for that cormorant and our troops and all the people being bombed. I wish I could errupt like a volcano to equal the violence and horror. The rage inside me has been frozen for so long.

Reheated by the immediate experience of fury at the war's massacre of the innocents, this woman made a dance in one therapy session that began to mediate her rage into consciousness (Perera 1988). She later named it "red-fire volcano against all destroyers."

Regression

Some individuals were forced to regress through layers well below shadow confrontation and the depressive position into paranoid-schizoidal processes and primary autism. They collapsed into what Wilfred Bion calls "psychotic crisis" where catastrophic change arouses feelings of disaster in participants and abruptly and violently subverts the order of things (Grinberg et al. 1977, p. 41). Many felt shame to find their usual sense of identity so dismembered by uncontained, overwhelming emotions as they suffered the "nameless dread" triggered by the war images. The reopening of aboriginal chaos, which came about through identification with the war images, evoked archetypal emotions: rage at overwhelming helplessness and uncontainment, anguish at abandoning loss, and terror for one's bodily integrity (Stewart 1986, p. 200).

The current experiences related to the war were intensified by and restimulated affects and experiences that had been palpably present and unmediated in very early childhood. For some clients, the outer chaos and the powerful images of war forced a sudden dismembering regression to what had been safely scarred over with primary defenses of denial, depersonalization, dissociation, projective identification, and splitting and framed into habitual character structures. Viewing the war images returned these analysands to levels of psyche and affect that revealed traumatic stresses in the parental/child complex, stresses so severe in some cases that they had prevented adequate learning about the process of metabolization of raw affects and about the creation of an incarnation vessel or ego center of consciousness that had the strength and integrity to survive and thrive.

The induction into what is a "realistic" madness is awful, but in some cases individuals were able to wrest from it a purpose and meaning. The overwhelming power of archetypal affects and presymbolic thoughts that were aroused by and hung projectively onto video images enabled some clients to experience a chronic psychosis that they could not experience in childhood, because they lacked then a viable container in which to confront such overwhelming anxiety. Adequate caretakers were not available to validate, protect against, or dose the overwhelming anxiety. Without adequate consciousness of self from which to disidentify and witness without unbearable pain, they had to withdraw instead behind various autistic and paranoid-schizoidal defenses (Ogden 1989, p. 102). They functioned in the world with only a brittle false self or persona. Now, in therapy, these analysands could use the therapeutic relationship as a container for the dismembering affects that blasted ego boundaries and opened consciousness into suffering the seemingly limitless space of chaos itself. Held within the transference and assisted by the analyst's empathy and countertransference awareness, they could begin to look beyond the emerging bizarre images and dismembering emotions for long-hidden personal memories. Within the constancy of analysis and by relying on the functioning aspects of their adult selves, these analysands could begin to use the regression to the psychotic part of themselves as the beginning of a healing process.[6]

Often collective and/or personal situations or relationships can restimulate and then begin to release the grip of fearful, traumatic

events and complexes by triggering or throwing us back into them in a
different context. Most often in therapy the transference and countertransference serves this function. It unsettles the inert, complacent
structures and defenses in which we habitually and blindly dwell and
forces us into psychological areas that still hold experiences of pain,
fears of the unknown, and boundless primal chaos. At this depth, we
must follow the guiding Self as we grope to understand our complexes
and express their energies in structures that may be more appropriate
for our individuation. This is slow, patient work. Sometimes, as with
this war, an outer event crashes through to the cellar, ripping open the
central complex like the SCUD/Patriot missile debris. From this violent
confrontation, we may begin to build a "new world order," but it is not
a simple Bushian concept to be bandied about to quell anxiety. It is
quite a perilous undertaking that involves us in a plunge into the
depths of our psychic wounds, into the maternal-child archetype with
its inchoate presymbolic fears of chaos, annihilation, and primary
affects, into what is madness and the still-remaining layers of madness
that are too often part of collective human culture. "War and madness
are scarcely unrelated," Michael Eigen says pointedly (1986, p. 20).

Toward Healing

The relatively well functioning woman who wrote about the chaos
of the first bombing of Baghdad soon recognized the analogies
between outer events and her inner madness. Plunged into preverbal
emotionality, she initially could not write or even express her mixed
emotions. She told me her mind was taken over by the incoherence of
primitive chaos. She said she had felt "blank terror and jittery, dissolving and all atremble." At first, like a psychotic, she felt uncertain of
boundaries and distinctions (inside/outside, animate/inanimate,
subject/object, image/meaning). She, therefore, could not feel that
she had a container for her chaotic reactions and could do nothing with
them except "sob like an infant overwhelmed." Disoriented, she hung
onto her friends and was only relieved of the "pressure of the bizarre"
when they could empathize with her, as they were also transfixed by the
television news. When her experience was thus validated, she could put
her extreme reactions into the collective emotional container—much as
an infant would put her anguish into the maternal-child field. Soothed
by the empathic mirroring of her friends, which she had rarely felt in
childhood with borderline parents, this woman could begin to experience herself as a more intact and open person responding to legitimate

horror. She could begin to disidentify from the outer events that reverberated into her wounded maternal-child complex and that dropped her into the pit of rearroused experiences of raw explosive primary emotions. She could even recognize that only part of her was swamped. The rest of her could hold, function, wash dishes, and even begin to hope that she could sort and metabolize an experience that felt so peculiarly shattering.

Later, alone, when the stress began to intensify again, she showed me that she had found another container for her reactions. She drew the chaos she felt in wild shapes and colors. Still later she tried to describe her "horrible jumble" by writing in her journal. Human empathy, art, and verbal expression all functioned as containers in which presymbolic chaos could be shaped into symbolic forms, providing some measure of control and disidentification. Finally she brought her journal and her still frighteningly ungrounded panic into analysis, allowing another level to be held for further exploration. Supported by the analyst's knowledge of her history, she began to realize that she was particularly susceptible to "night bombing," because her infancy had been marked by the explosions of a violently loud and insecure father returning from his late night workaholism to disrupt her sleep. Her mother had been unable to deal with the abusive sounds or to mediate her daughter's fear and protect her from the onslaught of archetypal emotion. Again, without shield and container, as the images of Desert Storm plunged into her peaceful consciousness, her early situation was replicated precisely, and she found an opportunity to explore her early body memories and to find mediating channels for her experience. She knew *about* her early fear and its effect on problems of sleeplessness and occasional paranoia; she had worked on these issues in analysis and body therapy. But she had not had any precise and forceful life trigger to bombard her with fear comparable to that which she knew as a child. The bombs falling on Baghdad served to create an uncanny replication of her infant emotions. Her friends, her art and journal, and her analysis validated her anxiety and helped her to contain and metabolize it. None of this had happened in her infancy. As a result, she had to bury her experiences of disaster in a closet of uncontained, nameless dread that was not to be fully reopened. Because she had looked through the crack several times before, she was able to endure the replication of her early experience relatively easily when the door of the forbidden room was blasted down. With that explosion, a new level of healing could begin.

Similarly the man terrified of terrorists was astonished to find that, rather than forcing him to face his fear of annihilation concretely as his parents had done by leaving him with abusive caretakers, his therapist supported his staying home in safety and using painting and dancing to express or "evacuate" his painful emotions and using the telephone for frequent therapy sessions. When the war hostilities ended and he felt able to risk the journey, he expressed a feeble and ashamed wish to take a friend along for the first trip rather than to brave the terrorist's den alone. The therapist—now an ambivalent object that both "forced" and protected the trip—still supported his need for safety. By validating and containing his terror through exploring its objective rationality, its need for nonverbal and verbal containers, and its roots in personal history and the transference, his therapy supported his actual safety and provided a multiple-leveled environment in which to explore and experience his psychotic fear in a new context. In an ensuing dream, he imaged himself riding in the elevator that had a floor, unlike earlier dreams in which floors were often missing. Rather than falling helplessly into an abyss of terror that he had felt and learned to deny in childhood, he discovered a safe-enough container for the human sensitivities that had been so abused. For this analysand, as for others, the war image riveted emotional attention to the psychotic pocket that was ready to open. Therapy then provided a concrete means of confronting, containing, and metabolizing the exposed chaotic elements. Previously this client had relied on sadistic superego categories to control his life and contain his emotions. He had also used denial, distancing, and dispersion of affect to manage eruptive lability and the underlying existential fear of annihilation.

As we can see in some analysands, Desert Storm unleashed a primordial sense of chaos and catastrophe. This chaos the Greeks imaged as the egg from which all life emerged. The alchemists called it the *prima materia*. This state is similar to the underlying sense of catastrophe which Bion saw as the matrix of the personality. For Bion, the primordial terror of this level links the parts of our personality together. For him, our first thoughts ("beta elements" made up of feelings of depression, persecution, guilt, envy) are indistinguishable from body sensations and float like hallucinations without a clear sense of boundaries and order. We try to expel these fragments to feel whole. Jungians would also call this primal level the *pleroma*—the primordial matrix of all that comes into existence. The pleroma is also the oblivion into which we redissolve consciousness in mystical experiences and in death. Most of our forms of awareness seem to violate this pleromatic boundlessness, because we usually know ourselves only as separate entities bounded within containing limits we feel are relatively safe—of body, family, group, locale, species, etc. We habitually use modes of consciousness that make us feel distinctions. In the West, we tend to identify ourselves with our limits and the verbal labels that express such closed forms.

Our dominant religious traditions have mythologized what we call earthly life as a Fall into matter and limited form. But they nonetheless posit the existence of another, more fluid realm in another dimension of time/space. Their images thus mediate the relationship between pleroma and closed forms. Modern science is closer to gnostic mystical traditions. It mythologizes an ocean of life energy that pervades all individual forms and species. Lacking experience of new paradigms of consciousness and a more permeable ego that are congruent with this worldview, we are too often personally caught in old formulations. We may then feel our lives permeated by dread of catastrophic submergence in the boundless sea that surrounds it. The burden falls on individual human caretakers, who are given the incompleted cultural task of mediating the transitions from pleromatic to limited, from unconsciousness to waking. Individuals carrying such an immense cultural task are inevitably inadequate. But they also provide the uncomfortable seedbeds of the new consciousness. Their very inadequacy forces the growth of new patterns of relationship between energy and form. Just because these early caretakers can rarely adequately and empathically mediate what the culture itself cannot bridge, vulnerable human infants are left to experience transitions from states of blissful fusion to separateness with a lurch of fear that must be managed by a primitive psyche that pulls in and away from others.

Such liminal spaces are filled with "beta elements" and primary emotions, and we may—in our psychotic parts—dread disintegration or dissolving in them. Or we may jump across from one emotion to another in our borderline parts, or we may pull away and repress our emotions into shadow areas if we are more neurotic. My sense is that we may do all of these, for we are formed in different layers like the snowflakes. Nonetheless, in early childhood times of greatest vulnerability, the patterns of dissolving, separating, bonding, and limiting are set. And we live with those patterns relatively unconsciously, dealing with experience according to inertial habits we may rarely even notice. As we have seen repeatedly, images of war serve to break through these inertial habits and open some individuals again to the experiences of chaos which formed them as they know themselves. Different psychological aspects are touched, but for some, these war images force them to return to face again the threat of death and the nameless dread that ushered them into life. They open us to the possibility of vastly enlarged and less rigidly fearful consciousness and even of transformation. They force us back to the fearsome matrix of life and consciousness from which any regeneration must come.

The Morrigan — Archetypal Images Behind War and Madness

Seeking an image of the matrix as the Mother of All Battles that could help to structure, hood, and give meaning to my own emotions about the war and with these clients' chaos, I thought of the various battling goddesses of heaven and earth. Many of these seemed too identified with active yang force, the energy of fighting itself. The patterns of energy that are made conscious in the archetypal images of Anath, Durga, Kali, Inanna, Maeve, Sekhmet, and Scathach did not mirror my clients' experiences or my own. The reactions I heard and felt to this war went to a more primeval level, one I associate to the raw images of the triad that the Irish called the Morrigan, the Mother of Life and of Death. She does not take part in battle as do many other goddesses, for the archaic culture out of which her stories grew has it roots deeper than the heroic period.

One man's dream, triggered by his experience of the Gulf War, presents an image that replicates one that we find in the ancient Irish tale, "The Cattle Raid of Regamna" or "Cu Chulainn and the Morrigan." The dream image is, in Bion's terms, a "bizarre object" (Grinberg et al. 1977, pp. 29ff):

Dream: *I am in my childhood house watching the war news on CNN. I suddenly see on the screen two people with a hobbyhorse monster. It's a pole with a head on it. Somehow I know that it is a person destroyed, without skin or flesh, just a pole and a red, bloody disk head. I scream with terror because it is also in the room.*

This analysand's childhood psychosomatic symptoms of intestinal cramps and diarrhea had reappeared with the onset of the war. Every morning, he awoke seized with painful spasms. While investigating the symptom medically, he also began to realize its psychological import: he felt unable to stomach or contain the stream of destructive and painful emotions by which he felt barraged. After affirming the horror of the war news and his somatic reactions, we also looked reductively for the circumstances in childhood that had initially elicited such symptoms. He began to perceive the degree of underlying existential fear that had gripped him all his life in reaction to which he had heroically proven himself by becoming a leader in his profession.

The skewered, puppetlike animal shows us the carrier of the life process as a monstrous, suffering distortion. In Jungian work, we also look for amplificatory material, which the Irish tale below provides. With it, we will now consider the archetype behind chaos and our defenses against it, behind the catastrophic experiences and images of psychosis and war, and behind the wisdom of suffering and bountiful life that may help to take us beyond madness and war. In the beginning of that tale:

When Cu Chulainn lay asleep in Dum Imrith, he heard a cry sounding out of the north, a cry terrible and fearful to his ears. Out of a deep slumber, he was aroused by it so suddenly that he fell out of his bed upon the ground like a sack, in the east wing of the house.

He rushed forth without weapons, until he gained the open air, his wife following him with his armor and garments. He perceived Loeg in his harnessed chariot coming towards him from . . . the North. "What brings thee here?" said Cu Chulainn.

"A cry that I heard sounding across the plain," said Loeg. . . .

"Let us follow the sound," said Cu Chulainn.

They went as far as Ath de Ferta (Ford of the Two Chariot Poles). When they arrived there, they heard the rattle of a chariot from the loamy district of Culgaire. They saw before them a chariot harnessed with *a chestnut horse. The horse had but one leg, and the pole of the chariot passed through its body so that the peg in front met the halter passing across its forehead.* Within the chariot sat a woman, [the Morrigan] her eyebrows red and a crimson mantle around her. Her mantle fell behind her between the wheels so that is swept along the ground. A big man went along beside the chariot. He also wore a coat of crimson, and on his back he carried a forked staff of hazelwood, while he drove a cow before him. (italics added)

The skewered, living hobbyhorse represents the motive power of the terrible goddess. The tale continues to reveal more about her:

"The cow is not pleased to be driven on by thee," said Cu Chulainn.

"She does not belong to thee," said the woman; "the cow is not owned by any of thy friends or associates."

"The cows of Ulster belong to me," said Cu Chulainn.

"Thou wouldst give a decision about the cow!" said the woman. "You are taking too much upon yourself, O Cu Chulainn!"

The mightiest of Ulster's warriors is made helpless before the Morrigan, and Cu Chulainn feels himself confused and ashamed. He then "made a leap into the chariot. He put his two feet upon her two shoulders and his spear on the parting of her hair." Undisturbed the woman orders him to move further off and recites a poem which only further frustrates him. When the warrior is about to spring again into the chariot, he finds that:

horse, woman, chariot, man and cow, all had disappeared. Then he perceived that she had been transformed into a black bird on a branch close by him. "A dangerous enchanted woman you are!" said Cu Chulainn. . . .

"If I had only known that it was thou," said Cu Chulainn, "we should not have parted thus."

"Whatever thou hast done," said she, "will bring thee ill luck."

"Thou canst not harm me," said he.

"Certainly I can," said the woman. "I am guarding thy deathbed, and I shall be guarding it henceforth."

The Morrigan tells him that the cow she leads came out of a fairy mound and that she is taking it to breed with the Bull of Cooley. She prophesies: "As long as her calf shall be a yearling, so long shall thy life be; and it is this that shall cause the Cattle-Raid of Cooley." The hero boasts of all the feats he will accomplish and the honor he will gain in that battle, and she reminds him that she will come against him:

"when thou art engaged in combat with a man as strong, as victorious, as dextrous, as terrible, as untiring, as noble, as brave, as great as thyself. I will become an eel, and I will throw a noose round thy feet in the ford so that heavy odds will be against thee."

"I swear by the god by whom the Ulstermen swear," said Cu Chulainn, "that I will bruise thee against a green stone of the ford; and thou shalt never have any remedy from me. . . ."

The Morrigan foretells that she will also attack the hero in the shape of a grey wolf that "will take strength from thy right hand, as far as to thy left arm." Cu Chulainn swears he will spear out her eye. Undeterred, the goddess promises she will then become a white, red-eared heifer who will lead a rush of [otherworldly] cows to trample him. He swears to break her legs (Cross and Slover 1936, pp. 211–214).

In another tale, we learn the outcome of the story. The hero is exhausted after his successful battle against his adversary and the animal shapes of the goddess. The Morrigan, in the shape of an old woman milking a cow with three teats, gives the exhausted hero milk. He blesses her and unknowingly heals the wounds he has inflicted on her when she shapeshifted into wolf, eel, and heifer (Kinsella 1970, pp. 135–137). Although the hero and the death goddess are adversaries, they are also related in another way, forever linked by mutual need (Neumann 1955, pp. 301ff).

We know the Morrigan best in other guises. Morgana le Fay of Avalon, who is King Arthur's sister and lover and a witch, is a later and tamer version. So is the elderly Lady Morgane who tested Sir Gawain through her son-in-law, the Green Knight. Older mythological evidence of the ancient Morrigan as a Great Goddess of the Irish is scattered throughout various medieval texts and in stories about parallel figures in Scotland, Gaul, and Wales. Her likeness is also represented in some Celtic relief sculptures. Gathering these bits, we can build a picture of this archetypal figure.

Old material tells of the Morrigan as a beautiful woman with nine loose tresses, washing herself on Samain, the New Year, at the fording place of the river. She has one foot on each side of the broad rushing torrent, straddling the waters of life. There she meets with the father god of the tribe when he comes to her for the destined sacred marriage rite of the New Year. The Morrigan was a pre-Celtic goddess of nature representing the inexhaustible process of life, death, and transformation. We can surmise that she was originally celebrated as the flowing rivers and bountiful and withholding earth. Mountains in Ireland are called her paps (breasts). She is often represented by cows. She is also depicted in stories by those most ancient of animal forms connected with the Great Goddess. We find her as snake, bird, mare, and wolf as well as feisty heifer and bountiful cow.

We find her presence manifest in myth on Samain (our Halloween), the Neolithic feast marking the end of the summer year, the end of the year king's life, and the beginning of the winter year. This goddess appears at liminal times—not only on Samain but also on the days of battle, death, or birth and in places like the fording shallows of the river when and where the boundaries between supernatural and natural worlds are thinnest, and the dead and living may pass readily to show the interpenetration of realms. The goddess represents the fated crossing from one realm to another as well as the wisdom that knows such crossings. Thus, she is the psychopomp of an ineluctable process.

The later lore of the Iron Age was patriarchal. In Celtic, aristocratic warrior stories written down by Christian scribes, such as the one above, the triune Nature Goddess was redefined and cast in a negative light. The name Morrigan came to connote both an individual goddess and the collective term to designate any of the "sinister, powerful and clearly ancient" triad of sisters or supernatural beings who haunt the battlefields (Ross 1967, p. 223). As death and battle goddesses, these were said to influence events by magic and by inspiring terror in the hearts of warriors. They are associated with various destructive animals and made into hags. Nonetheless, they retained their marked sexual and fertility characteristics. The Morrigan in the chariot with her red eyebrows and sweeping red cloak is served by a herdsman, who drives her cow. Although she is ruler of death and fate, she remains the nurturing cow goddess. In this story, she chides Cu Chulainn, the guardian of the Ulster tribe and its herds, for taking too much upon himself by claiming her cow.

Many ancient goddesses appear in triune form. Sometimes these were differentiated as maiden, mother, and hag. The Morrigan, however, is a more primordial triad, one interwoven and relating to her shapeshifts between different levels of consciousness. She is differentiated into the Morrigan, Nemain, Badb, and sometimes Macha instead of Nemain. The first of the triad, and the name of the whole group is the Morrigan, Great Queen or Queen of Demons. She appears in various animal and human shapes including that of a beautiful seductress who lures the hero to herself. More often she appears as a nurturing or loathesome hag. In our story, she is not as visibly ugly as in some others, but when the warrior Cu Chulainn asks for her own and her companion's identities, she pours out a string of nearly unintelligible nonsense words interspersed with more threatening names: "cold wind," "cutting," and "terror" (Sjoestedt 1982, p. 48).

The Morrigan appears in the story "The Destruction of Da Derga's Hostel" as huge and hideous. It is again Samain, the night of an inevitable terrible raid and the king's death. She arrives first with a henchman who is carrying a roasted pig that is still squealing — another one of the bizarre images that the Celts used to convey the paradox of death in life and fertile life in death. She is described as "huge, black, gloomy, big-mouthed, [and] ill-favored" with a snout that a branch might support and lower lips (or pudenda) extending to her knees. Later:

in the hostel, [this] woman appeared at the entrance, after sunset, and sought to be let in. As long as a weaver's beam, and as black, her two shins. She wore a very fleecy, striped mantle. Her beard reached her knees, and her mouth was on one side of her head. She put one shoulder against the doorpost and cast a baleful eye upon the king and the youths about him, and Conare [the king] said to her from inside the house, "Well then, woman, what do you see for us, if you are a seer?" "Indeed, I see that neither hide nor hair of you will escape from this house, save what the birds carry off in their claws," the woman replied. "It is not ill fortune that we prophesied, woman," said Conare. "Neither do you usually prophesy for us. What is your name?" "Cailb," she replied.[7] "A name with nothing to spare that," said Conare. "Indeed, I have many other names," she said. . . . [and she] recited [thirty-one of] these in one breath, and standing on one foot, at the entrance of the house. (Gantz 1981, p. 76)

The names include the festival, Samuin, the river, Shannon, the Irish words for "panic," "horror," and "scald crow" as well as many nonsense words — perhaps remnants of a magical invocation and/or suggestions of the bewildering cognitive chaos this goddess brings with her.

Again in "Da Choca's Hostel" she is described with comparable hideousness as a . . . big-mouthed, black, swift, sooty woman, lame and squinting with her left eye. She wore a threadbare dingy cloak. Dark as the back of a stag beetle was every joint of her, from the top of her head to the ground. Her filleted grey hair fell back over her shoulder. She leant her shoulder against the

doorpost and began prophesying evil to the host, and to utter ill words. . . .
then the Badv went from them. (Ross 1967, p. 248)

Her hideous anthropomorphic form evokes the horror of violent
destruction to come. Unlike the hag in other Celtic (and Vedic) myths,
who can be disenchanted by a brave partner's kiss, the Morrigan stands
apart and seems to bring only "ill fortune" or "evil" to her heroic
partners. In only one remaining tale, after making love with a divine
partner, the father god of the Tuatha pantheon, does she bring help
and favorable advice (Cross and Slover 1936, pp. 38–39). Usually she
foretells and initiates mortals into the unknown state that we call
death. It is our fear of annihilation that is projected onto her as loathe-
someness. The experience of change seems like a death. Dying as the
process of crossing into what is unknown and still unconscious seems
only malefic and monstrous to the individual identified with present
consciousness. The Morrigan is thus haglike and monstrous because her
power over our inevitable and destined end is seen only negatively as
the finality of death in a world that has lost connection to the cyclic and
transformative process she represents.[8] Yet today we are again redefin-
ing our relationship to the unknown and unconscious by revaluing
many forms of awareness that render them more accessible to us.[9] Our
sense of identity and consciousness is expanding to include forms of
awareness that render "ego" more permeable and closer to the Self just
as the ego's tightly edged boundaries are being stretched to include the
experienced reality of more process-oriented modalities and even of the
dissolutions and reformings that feel like death and regeneration. We
are finding that it is only by overcoming our fear of going through the
many changes in our development demanded by the Self that the new
ego—one in tune with the Self's guidance—can emerge. Like the sha-
manic warriors of old who had to learn to live with death as a constant
companion, so we need to practice and struggle to overcome the fears
that make us shrink back into defensive securities that render us inert.
Through time and the many deaths we experience in our development,
we may gain a sense of the "me" that is able to flow or lurch or
scramble, even kicking and screaming, to serve the Self's intent.

Fate and Destiny

Typically the Morrigan is a figure of fate and the female wisdom of
serpent, raven, and flowing waters, and blood. As birthing, destroying,
and regenerating aspects of the whole life process, she represents sight
from the pleromatic perspective—the cosmic eye, which sees from the

matrix underlying and beyond opposites, uniting what is below and above, past and future, the snake's and bird's eye views. Like the triple Norns who "rise out of the ground with the spring of living water, knowing both Life and Death" (Herzog 1966, p. 97), she is thus the prophet of destiny. She can foretell the outcome of the battles of life to those who ask. Even today, rites of divination take place at Samain, the night on which the ancient Celtic kings must die and the new cycle begins.

Sometimes the Morrigan is depicted at the crossing of the water, washing the armor and weapons of those about to be slain in battle. In the story "Da Choca's Hostel," King Cormac and his men see a red woman standing in the water of the ford washing the cushions and harness of a chariot. When she lowers her hand, the riverbed becomes red with blood and gore. When she raises it, the water also rises and leaves the riverbed dry so an army might cross easily. Repulsed by the sight of her, the king asks one of his men to approach the hag and ask what she is going there. Standing in the magician's ritual posture—on one foot, with one hand raised, and one eye open, to represent the unity of the cosmic perspective, she chants that she is washing the arms of the doomed king (Ross 1967, p. 245). With such foreknowledge, he must still carry on bravely—as we all must. The magician's pose in which the goddess stands is typical in Irish tradition. It conveys the idea of energy roused to the pitch of intensity that provides power for magical intent. Monocular, single-pointed, preambivalent energy holds an orgiastic potential that has effective power in the magic dimension of consciousness to focus emotion and compel events. Such focused energy provides a powerful tool of magic in the occult traditions. The posture gives us an apt image for the seemingly magical compulsion of split affect states that we may experience—often by induction—generated from borderline levels of the psyche.

In the myth "The Tain," the Cattle Raid of Cooley, the Morrigan again foretells the outcome of events, but she also acts to rouse the bull force to participate in the destined events of battle. The text says she "settled in bird shape on a standing stone" and sang to the Brown Bull—the totem of the armies of the north. She describes the anxiety that will mount before the fight and the beautiful land in its prosperous bounty that is doomed to destruction. As the sinister force behind life and death, she sings the stark contrast of bounty and death (good breast and bad) in a poem that expresses how many of us felt last winter as war preparations in the Persian Gulf intensified:

> Dark one are you restless
>   do you guess they gather
> to certain slaughter
>   the wise raven
> groans aloud
>   that enemies infest
> the fair fields
>   ravaging in packs
> learn   I descern
>   rich plains
> softly wavelike
>   baring their necks
> greenness of grass
>   beauty of blossoms
> on the plains war
>   grinding heroic
> hosts to dust
>   cattle groans the Badb
> the raven   ravenous
>   among corpses of men
> affliction and outcry
>   and war everlasting
> raging over Cuailnge
>   death of sons
> death of kinsmen
>   death   death!
> (Kinsella 1970, p. 98)

With this terrible dirge, the Morrigan rouses the bull to participate in the dire process that returns all that thrives to the abyss through grinding, devouring death.

Before the famous second battle of Moyatura, which is part of the mythic history of Ireland, the Morrigan trysts with the father god of the Tuatha De Danann. Then she helps him by providing information of the enemy landings and a present of two handfuls of her own sacred blood, which streams forth in birth and battle to deprive the foe of "the blood of his heart, and the kidneys of his valor."[10] As the spirit of war, she "heartened the Tuatha De to fight the battle fiercely and fervently" until the battle becomes a rout. Then after the battle was won and the corpses cleared away, the Morrigu proceeded to proclaim that battle and mighty victory which had taken place, to the royal heights of Ireland and to its fairy hosts and its chief waters and its rivermouths. And hence it is that Badb (i.e., the Morrigu) also describes high deeds. (Cross and Slover 1936, p. 45)

The Morrigan is one singer of the gods, the voice of fate in which we may find our own stories. And these stories inevitably express alternations and ambivalence — moments of triumph followed by collapse, moments of order followed by chaos, and vice versa. The Morrigan sings one song that is redolent with the bounty of life and the process by which things attain their peaceful order. She sings to celebrate the end of a war:

> Peace up to heaven,
> Heaven down to earth,
> Earth under heaven,
> Strength in every one. . . .

The images lure us to relax just as we did after the fighting in the Persian Gulf seemed to bring peace. But our experience of Desert Storm is echoed in the Morrigan's song. The old text immediately shatters our comfort and unsettles any security we might crave. It continues by telling us:

Then moreover, she was prophesying the end of the world, and foretelling every evil that would be therein, and every disease and every vengeance. Wherefore she sang this lay:

> "I shall not see a world that will be dear to me.
> Summer without flowers,
> Kine will be without milk,
> Women without modesty,
> Men without valor,
> Captures without a king. . .
> Woods without mast,
> Sea without produce. . . .
> Wrong judgments of old men,
> False precedents of lawyers,
> Every man a betrayer,
> Every boy a reaver.
> Son will enter his father's bed.

Father will enter his son's bed,
Every one will be his brother's brother-in-law. . . .
An evil time!
Son will deceive his father,
Daughter will deceive her mother."
(Cross and Slover 1936, p. 48)

The new world order seemingly established by victory is destroyed by the turbulence that inevitably follows. Peaceful bounty gives way to infertility; social stability gives way to chaos in society and incest in the family. Disruption overturns the previously ordered forms to force life forward in an endless rhythmic process. So after our momentary victory in Iraq, Kurds are dying, more refugees are fleeing, oil wells are seething black flames and soot across the sky, mysterious plagues kill the survivors. There is more starvation, more homelessness, more pollution and nuclear proliferation, more disillusionment. Like the river whose force she represents, the Morrigan warns us in this poem that human life appears to be a series of chaotic, rapid drops in the flow. In her grim view, stasis, triumph, and peace appear as only little pools of momentary safety and/or inertia in the flow that rises and falls with the seasons and the currents of its larger matrix. War, chaos, and abrupt flux between the pools predominate. Such is the sight and song of the Morrigan's vision. It challenges us to find ways other than those of war's upheavals to create and sustain change.

Shapeshifter

Moving from one perspective to the other as a seer and singer of the life process, the Morrigan is also a shapeshifter. In our story of Cu Chulainn and the Morrigan, the red-browed hag shapeshifts into a raven, a bird form with which she is often associated. Then she is called by the name of the second goddess in the triad, Badb (crow), the raven or crow of battle. Sometimes the goddess Morrigan or Badb is also represented as a devouring wolf. Raven and wolf are viscerally gripping images of the matrix that dissolves or, more aptly here, devours all life forms back into itself. When the storytellers of the warrior aristocracy want to suggest that the goddess's powers are unimportant to the real hero, they sing of the mighty Mac Cecht, who "was among the wounded on the field of slaughter." This great warrior complains with typically heroic bravado that something like a fly or midge is nipping at his fatal wound. A woman, passing through the slaughterfield (and she may even be another form of the Morrigan herself) honors the old powers with her deeper and wider view. With empathic "fear and horror" at the carnage around her, she renames what the stoic hero calls a little midge, telling him that it is the wolf that is already gnawing his bloodied body. She calls the wolf an "ant of the ancient earth" (Gantz 1981, p. 105). With this metaphor, she evokes the Morrigan's powers to clean up the carrion left from battle. She calls on the goddess as eater of the dead, who buries broken forms back into her bowels and re-earths the fallen hero. In Irish tales, the battlefield itself is called "the garden of Badb" (Sjoestedt 1982, p. 45), for the dead are both the harvest of the death goddess and her seed food, dying into the earth for regeneration.

Thus, when Badb appears in human form, she has a marked sexual character—a huge vulva like the Sheila-na-gigs and is also associated with the rites of childbirth. Badb, the raven, was also considered a psychopomp, carrying off the dead in her claws to the otherworld, like the Norse Valkyries and Indian dakinis who were said to claim the final breath of the dying with a kiss of peace. An old pagan song contains these words:

> Fear not, the raven's red eye,
> Her sight all aflaming will shine on our hearts.
> Fear not, the raven's black wing,
> The light of her feathers will carry us home. . . .

Sometimes the third of the Morrigan triad is Nemain. From the wider, pleromatic perspective, she represents the ritualized shamanlike possession that the Celts sought in order to experience predifferentiated atonement with all forms of life. This totally open state of *participation mystique* allows us to experience ecstatic fusion with the underlying matrix of life and attain perception of the essence of discrete life forms. It provides a wisdom that is beyond common sense and science as it is currently practiced. This ecstatic and mystical vision is related to the "radical presence" of ecological consciousness that we are struggling to reawaken in our culture (Macy 1991, p. 36). It is an affect-based correlate of what Jung calls "absolute knowledge."

But from the perspective of the combative warriors, Nemain is the frenzy of battle madness that sweeps them into combat with violent excitement, a state the Romans identified with the Celts and called the "*Furor Gallicus*." Nemain literally means frenzy or panic. This ecstatic possession by rage made the Celts intrepid and fearsome adversaries, who rushed headlong into battle, naked except for the neck torc that bound them to their deity. They were filled with the inebriation of the war goddess as a raging frenzy, like a psychotic rage that can totally possess those seized by it. Panic is the other side of frenzy. It represents a mad seizure by terror in response to the uncontrollable forces that possess us. In contrast to the passion to fight that represents the drive to defend our more coherent sense of self, Nemain's panic makes us go mad, dissociate, or even die. Instead of fighting wildly, we flee. One story tells us that Nemain once used her power to rouse panic in the enemy "and confusion in the army so that the four provinces of Ireland massacred each other with their own spears and their own weapons, and that a hundred warriors died of terror and heart-failure that night" (Kinsella 1970, p.223).

This primordial aspect of the Morrigan is similar to the wild and nameless dread that assails us when we are confronted by our own helplessness before the vast forces of life and death. It may be the terror we endure as we are buffeted through the birth canal to confront life outside the womb, lacking strength, coordination, and even adequate myelin sheathing for raw nerves. We may meet this dread again many times in life before the onslaught of any severe trauma. Some people found such dread stirred by images of Desert Storm. The nearly inchoate and threatening words by which the Morrigan names herself aptly evoke this sense of primordial terror that we suffer in the grip of catastrophe — nonsense words (like Bion's beta elements) interspersed with threatening allusions to "cold wind," "cutting," and "terror." Nemain represents the imageless, dread-filled emptiness or chaos of the *prima materia* — an experience we flee when we have felt overwhelming pains in infancy before we have coalesced a constant sense of other to trust and/or before we have coalesced a constant sense of ourselves to defend. It is in the face of this overwhelming terror that we are sometimes reduced to psychotic processes, which may safeguard us from our experience of fear by primitive hallucinations, mindlessness, dissolution or rigidity, hate, chaotic ideation, and reversals.

In our story, it is Nemain's dissolving cry that, like a nightmare, rouses the fearless Ulster warrior Cu Chulainn and sends him rushing out unclothed. The sound from the pleromatic abyss threatens to dissolve all boundaries that permit life forms to manifest. From the perspective of the pleroma, these forms are only illusions (like Maya in India), but they nonetheless give shape and substance to life on earth. It is their valued discreteness that the hero leaps out of unconsciousness to defend. As guardian of the Ulster tribe, his task is to preserve the sacred structures and boundaries that permit social discourse and cultural order. Fear can stimulate heroic aggression to defend those forms.

Comparable dread of the terrible matrix is what my analysand who dreamed of the hobbyhorse felt when he erupted into his childhood mornings with his stomach skewered in knots. In his life he had become a hero defending the boundaries and structures of conscious life. When we have known only horror within a terrible matrix, family container, or maternal relationship, we are frightened by the seeming threat of returning to any relationship in which we might feel dependent. Because we expect a repetition of early suffering, we use all our creativity to erect defenses against the presumed threat of such agony. The prospect of lowering habitual defensive consciousness and fusing with another may fascinate us, but it also propels us to flee and rigidify our grip on the defensive structures to which we cling. We try to stay vigilant. We may feel paranoid. We may leap eruptively into the intoxicating thrill of rage and battle, letting the excitement hold us like a surrogate mother.

We could also say that to the woman who feared the gas threat, the television images served her as Nemain's cry. They roused her out of mute and relatively peaceful denial to restimulate her inchoate terror of early entanglement in a destructively dissolving matrix. They aroused panicky flight reactions. Whether defended by fight or flight, the underlying fear of too early, too negative experience of the pleroma opened the psychotic pockets that so many people experienced under bombardment by the images of the war. Such dread itself has no image, for we originally felt it before we could manage our relation to images or hold even parts of them constant in memory. Such dread grips the gut. It seizes us from inside like Nemain's penetrating, horrible scream and makes us feel we are going to pieces. We feel we will fall forever, without relationship to the body and without orientation. These states call up what Winnicott named "unthinkable anxiety" (1965, p. 58). They are Nemain's realm. Only by returning regressively to experience these states as deeply wounded aspects of our infant/maternal bonding and by reexperiencing our fear of them in a different context can we even begin to heal and to find our own creativity freed. Whether such healing is at all possible and to what extent often seems more a matter of grace and destiny than clinical fit and skill. But in this imageless area of "unthinkable anxiety," the figure of Nemain herself gives us the gift of an image that can help immeasurably when dealing with our psychotic parts and their processes.

Sometimes the third of the Morrigan trio is Macha, the mare

goddess of life, agricultural prosperity, battle, and death. In Irish tales, she brings bounty to her chosen partners and tribespeople, sovereignty to her chosen kings, and glory to her warriors. The heads of the battle dead are like the heads of grain to the mare goddess. They are called "the mast [seed food] of Macha." In our story of Cu Chulainn and the Morrigan, the goddess's agricultural and battle steed is a bizarre, monstrous apparition like the weird, bloody hobbyhorse in the analysand's dream. Its appearance in Celtic lore is reminiscent of royal burial rites in several cultures. In Scythian royal funerals, Herodotus tells us, the finest horses were killed, disemboweled, stuff with chaff and stitched up with stakes run through them from neck to tail (Ross 1967, p. 222). Sacrificed to be literal psychopomps, they went into the tomb to carry their royal masters to the otherworld. Comparable impalements are found in Gaulish sacrificial customs and myths. One witness describes British Queen Boudicca's sacrifice of women before her tribe's victorious battle with the Romans who had raped her daughters and stolen her lands. He tells us that the women dedicated to the goddess Andraste had "their breasts cut off and stuffed in their mouths, so that they seemed to be eating them, then their bodies were skewered lengthwise on sharp stakes" (Cassius Dio, quoted by Ross 1967, p. 222). Andraste, like the Morrigan, represented the paradox of bounty and milk, war and destruction. Thus women sacrificed to her to arouse war energy had their breasts removed, indicating that nurturant energy was to be reassimilated to become available as (oral) aggression. As Lady Macbeth wished metaphorically to be, the women dedicated to the goddess were "unsexed" literalistically, mutilated to be rendered incapable of nurture and forced to assume a horrifying, aggressive form.

Usually we feel safe from the magic consciousness of such concretistic terrors. But when we are seized on the archaic level of the Morrigan, our dreams are as full of such gory stuff as were the ancient rites. How are we to process the "bizarre image" of the skewered one-legged horse? Are we to defend against its impact by distancing our consciousness from its horror, by labeling it as "collateral damage?" Are we to say such an image is "psychotic," pretending it is Other as if we do not all have roots in this layer of the psyche? Are we to frame it as an "interesting archetype" or label it "a witch's hobbyhorse" to drain its potency? Then we can deny and avoid any visceral empathy with the sadistically tortured, gruesome animal that represents a part of human experience.

This hideous image suggests that the ongoing process of life energy has been maimed, rigidly impaled, and staggers on only one leg. It is an image like that of the crucifixion but borne by the instinctual form of the mother who carries all life. Uncannily, in the myth, the horse moves on—like the cooked pig that squeals. Realistically it should be dead. This image aptly suggests the horror of maimed, rigidly impaled, and suffering life that underlies both war and psychosis. And if, like the man who dreamed of a similar horse, we have met such horror in our childhood house, it is no wonder his young body used diarrhea to lessen its grip and frantic masturbation to find some rigidly automatic, self-sufficient, heroic holding for himself. Too early and too personally, he had to face the unmediated experience of the suffering earth spirit in a monstrous revelation of life in death or destructive sadism in life.

Serpent

The analysand who was terrified of the chemical weapon's threat dreamed that she had taken "a bottle marked with spiral-coiled snakes from the [therapist's] office. Somehow it was able to contain the [deathly] gas." Working on the dream image, she began to recognize that there was a holding environment in therapy that could mitigate her fears of dissolving into vapor. She associated the snakes to the medical sign of healing, but they were not wound around a caduceus. I recognized the far older motif of the spirals of energy that mark many ancient sites and artifacts to suggest life's endless transformations. The snakes coiled around her dream bottle mark it as a vessel of the goddess's powers over life, death, and regeneration—a serpent power commensurate with the all-potent destructiveness that had been the terrorizing ruler of this woman's life—a ruler which she described as "Death, the familiar air of my childhood."

Such power was originally associated with the Great Goddess of the serpent rivers, the earth's energy lines, and the snake. The Morrigan, like the river's winding flow, was one of the primordial serpent goddesses of Neolithic Ireland (cf. Gimbutas 1989, pp. 121–124). Sometimes even called Lamia in text and on sculptures (Ross 1967, p. 223), the triple Morrigan resembles Middle Eastern serpent and bird goddesses like the pre-Hellenic Medusa/Athena (Walker 1983, p. 629). Indeed there are two tales linking the Morrigan to the ancient serpent goddess of the Celts. In one, her serpent form is changed to that of a water eel, which twines itself three times around Cu Chulainn's legs during one of his battles and drags him under the water to make him suffer defeat for spurning her (Kinsella 1970, p. 135). In the other, the Morrigan's serpent power is more totally negated, for the story expresses Christian repugnance for the ancient cult and shows us clearly what happened to pagan images of power and of the ecstatic interconnection and fullness of life.

In a legend connected with the Morrigan's son Meiche that explains the name of the River *Berbha* (Barrow), we read how the goddess's original power is projected and negated. Seen only as destructive, it still cannot be destroyed. The place-name legend asks "Whence *Berbha*, [Barrow]?" and then answers the question by telling us how the river got its name:

> Into this river were thrown the three snakes that were (found) in the heart of the Morrigan's son Meiche after he was slain by Diancecht [the healer god of the later and more patriarchal Tuatha pantheon] on Magh Meichi; which plain's name at first was Magh Fertaighe. The three hearts that were in Meiche bore the shape of three serpent's heads and, had not the killing of him come to pass, those snakes would have grown in his belly and eventually left no animals alive in Ireland. When he had slain Meiche, Diancecht burned the snakes and their ashes he committed to that current, with the effect that it seethed and boiled to rags all living things that were therein. (Ross 1967, pp. 345–356)

We know the triple goddess as a triple spiral of snakes from the carving deepest inside the great third-millenium B.C. mound temple at New Grange. In this much later place-name tale, the snakes are projected into the Great Goddess's son and denigrated as his three evil hearts. The serpent power of the waters of life and the spring river's warming was connected to many river goddesses and their healing cults. Here it is deprived of its connection to the feminine and to healing. It is reversed and negated, made into a one-sided power to destroy, leaving "no animals alive in Ireland." The story suggests the priests hoped that by teaching that their power was evil the snakes of the old religion might be driven out of Ireland and cut out of human hearts. Meiche, son of the Morrigan, becomes a killing dragon monster and devil. Severed from its place in the whole process of life's flow and burned to ash, the serpent power cannot be destroyed. Projected, reversed, denigrated, corrupted, and one-sided, it is still indestructible. Burned and dissolved, it maintains its potency, albeit now only destructively, by making the water seethe and turning the living to rags. The pagan healer god Diancecht, like the later snake-banisher, Saint Patrick, cannot fully repress what he brands as evil. His actions merely focus and potentize it. He cannot even destroy the remnants of the old religion, for the name of the Morrigan's son, although now identified only with destructive power, becomes the name of a grassy plain. And the river where the ash of his heart snakes was strewn is called Barrow. This name reminds us of the transformative process that reduces and carries away forms of life as if they were rags—just as the barrow mound raised as a tomb in Neolithic times carries us to dust and the otherworld, just as the barrow cart moves earth and its harvests and compost.

The ancient potency of the spiral marked the jar of the analysand's dream. We may experience its more one-sided negative and destructive form when we feel only the loss that any death brings. Then if we identify with the structure that is dissolving to rags, we fear the serpent power, because we cannot yet see the whole process that it symbolizes. In therapy, the chaos-making and corrosive powers of destruction appear to dissolve forms of relationship. Images of such negating powers may coincide with a phase of depression or negative transference or with a descent into chaos to free space and energy for new forms to emerge. Inevitably even images of good-enough containments and relationships may become negative to the analysand or child in order to make space for separation to discover new patterns more congruent with current development needs. During such inevitable phases (which sometimes feel like personal destruction), therapist and parent must suffer and abide through the destruction of the old bonds, seeking for trust in the larger process. This often includes letting go of defenses against the negative transference.

Raven

The Morrigan sometimes appears in raven form. As a black, noisy, ever-alert bird, the raven sounds alarm with her raucous cries and lives even in poetry as a forboding voice. She struts on the ground displacing smaller birds, a match even for small animals. Large and omnivorous, she sweeps down on the fields to eat both the grain of their harvest and any unburied carrion.[11] We read in an old text that the "longing" of the Irish crow or raven goddess was said to be for war, chaos, dismemberment:

> . . . for the fire of combat;
> The warrior's sides slashed open,
> Blood, bodies heaped upon bodies;
> Eyes without life, sundered heads,

> these are pleasing . . . to her.
> (D'Arbois 1970, p. 110)

Later folksongs of the three ravens who sat in a tree over a dead knight hearkens back to this triple goddess and her harvest. In the Celtic cult of the Raven Goddesses, black-robed women flapping like crows raced among the warriors to stir up their war frenzy before battle, just as the raven's song roused the Brown Bull. We know that the presence of these wild raven women among the Welsh at Anglesey roused fear in the Roman soldiers opposing them (A.D. 62).

In this cult, the three-fold raven goddess was honored by sacrifice. A description "imperfectly understood by those who committed the old oral tale to writing" in the early Middle Ages tells us of

a trio, naked, on the ridge-pole of the house: their jets of blood coming through them, and the ropes of slaughter on their necks. "Those I know" says [the speaker], "three of awful boding. Those are the three that are slaughtered at every time." (Ross 1967, p. 248)

The presence of the goddesses on the ridge-pole implies that they are in their bird form. The blood and hanging represent the sacrifice of birds in the cult—the goddess sacrificing to herself much as the Celtic-influenced raven god Odin did when he hung on his tree "given to Odin, myself to myself."

Just as she had predicted when she told him she was "guarding" his deathbed, "the battle goddess Morrigu and her sisters" came in raven shape to sit on the shoulders of the mortally wounded Cu Chulainn. Their presence informs his enemies that they had nothing more to fear from the quintessential hero, for his fated death had come upon him. As one of his thus heartened enemies said laconically before the hero was finally beheaded, "That pillar is not wont to be under birds" (Cross and Slover 1936, p. 338). Indeed all through his short life until he broke all his taboo and lost his strength, Cu Chulainn fended off the death the Morrigan had in store for him. Then she flew to his shoulder and claimed him finally as hers. Celtic heroes are termed those "who know the way of the black ravens," for warriors inevitably live closely with death, building their bravery, power, and fame in defending their lives against its pull and their own fear of disintegration.

The raven often appears in analysands' material to symbolize the dark energies and far-sightedness of the triple goddess. Representing the spirit devouring and/or carrying primordial libido, the raven usually signifies a transitional phase marking the process whereby, for example, manic defenses are opening into depression, depression is moving toward rage and curiosity, or rage-defended fear is shifting toward dependency. Representing the ideation of a dark vision of the otherworld, the raven destines and supports our crossing over such transitions. To make them, we inevitably return to the matrix that is both feared and needed in order to develop our integrity and capacity for interrelatedness. The image of the Morrigan represents annihilation, rage, death, birth, and regeneration in one whole that presents a nearly unbearable challenge to our consciousness. Thus, the Morrigan is connected to regression to the psychotic parts of us and to the terrible upheavals in the collective that we call war.

Conclusion

The Gulf War and its aftermath have indeed been traumatic on many levels. The images of war opened chaotic pockets even in those of us who were fortunate enough to be only participant observers. We find similar images in the mythologems surrounding the Celtic deity called the Morrigan. These horrific images hold up mirrors of the dread, dissolution, dismemberment, and rage that we may have experienced in the grip of unmediated primary affects. On the one hand, they are the projection of that misery discovered and created by the primary caretaker turned destroyer. On the other hand, they are the mirrors of what is always beyond us and threatening our sense of secure boundaries and secure identities. They provide images of the unknown that we dread, forcing us to "the great and ultimate task [that] is to understand fear in all its forms as an instrument of the Self" (Neumann 1986, p. 28). Such images provide terrifying and ravishing experiences of the pleromatic source. To individuate, these experiences of fear must be lived through—sometimes as psychotic episodes in which the adult can metabolize and transform what the infant could not bear and had to eject and/or deny. At other times, such experiences form the basis of spiritual crises in which the adult is forced to confront the Mother of All Battles, the matrix of chaos, fear, grief, rage, birth, bounty and mystic atonement with the macrocosm. Such working through is analogous to facing the fearful reality of the unconscious and coming to terms with what comes through the battles of life and the destruction of life forms and is also beyond these battles and destructions. As we struggle to work out new relationships to such seemingly chaotic and painful paradoxes—life in death and death in life—we may regain access to the polyvalent matrix that supports us. Subsequently from that ground of renewal, we may discover and create a new heroic stance and/or the wisdom of empathic consciousness and a capacity for blessing the very matrix from which we arise and in which we surrender.

References

Bernstein, Jerome S. 1989. *Power and Politics: The Psychology of Soviet-American Partnership*. Boston: Shambhala.

Cross, T. P., and Slover, C. H. 1936. *Ancient Irish Tales*. New York: Henry Holt and Co.

D'Arbois de Jubainville, H. 1903. *The Irish Mythological Cycle and Celtic Mythology*. R. I. Best, trans. New York: Lemma Publishing Co., 1970.

Eigen, Michael. 1986. *The Psychotic Core*. Northvale: Jason Aaronson Inc.

Gantz, Jeffrey. 1981. *Early Irish Myths and Sagas*. New York: Penguin Books.

Gimbutas, Marija. 1989. *The Language of the Goddess*. San Francisco: Harper and Row.

Grinberg, L., Sor, D. and Tabak de Bianchedi, E. 1977. *Introduction to the Work of Bion*. New York: Jason Aronson.

Hacker, Carol. 1991a. AMHCA responds to the traumas of Desert Storm. *The Advocate*, vol. 14, no. 6 (February).

Hacker, Carol. 1991b. AMHCA helps the healing of Desert Storm. *The Advocate*, vol. 14, no. 7 (March).

Herzog, Edgar. 1966. *Psyche and Death*. New York: G. P. Putnam and Sons.

Ierodiakonou, C. S. 1970. The effect of the threat of war on neurotic patients in psychotherapy. *American Journal of Psychotherapy* vol. 24, no. 4 (October).

Jung, C. G. 1949. *Letters I: 1906–1950*. G. Adler, ed. Princeton, N.J.: Princeton University Press, 1973.

Keen, Sam. 1986. *Faces of the Enemy: Reflections of the Hostile Imagination*. San Francisco: Harper and Row.

Kinsella, T. 1970. *The Tain*. London: Oxford University Press.

Macy, Joanna. 1991. Interview. *New Age Journal* (January-February), p. 36.

Neuman, Erich. 1955. *The Great Mother: An Analysis of the Archetype*. Princeton, N.J.: Princeton University Press.

————. 1952. The psyche and the transformation of the reality planes. *Spring* (1956), pp. 81–111.

————. 1986. Fear of the feminine. *Quadrant* 19, 1:7–30.

Ogden, Thomas H. 1989. *The Primitive Edge of Experience*. Northvale: Jason Aaronson.

Perera, Sylvia B. 1988. Ritual integration of aggression in psychotherapy. *The Borderline Personality in Analysis*, M. Stein and N. Schwartz-Salant, eds. Wilmette, Ill.: Chiron Publications, pp. 233–266.

Ross, Anne. 1967. *Pagan Celtic Britain: Studies in Iconography and Tradition*. London: Routledge and Kegan Paul.

Sjoestedt, Marie-Louise. 1982. *Gods and Heroes of the Celts*. Berkeley, Calif.: Turtle Island.

Stevens, Anthony. 1989. *The Roots of War: A Jungian Perspective*, New York: Paragon House.

Stewart, Louis H. 1986. Work in progress: affect and archetype: a contribution to a comprehensive theory of the structure of the psyche. *The Body in Analysis*, M. Stein and N. Schwartz-Salant, eds. Wilmette, Ill.: Chiron Publications, pp. 183–203.

Wagner, Rojean. 1991. The effects of war: war news may trigger depression, anxiety in some viewers. *The Psychiatric Times* 7(3).

Walker, Barbara G. 1983. *The Woman's Encyclopedia of Myths and Secrets*. San Francisco: Harper and Row.

Winnicott, Donald W. 1965. *The Maturational Processes and the Facilitating Environment:*

Studies in the Theory of Emotional Development. New York: International Universities Press.

Notes

1. In some sensitive individuals, the clinical symptoms of profound anxiety about the oncoming war cannot necessarily be attributed to paranoia and pessimism. It may be that certain individuals were intuiting this truth in spite of overt denials. On March 3, 1991, in the Sunday *New York Times,* Thomas L. Friedman and Patrick E. Tyler reported, in an article entitled "From the First, US Resolve to Fight," that the plans for an offensive campaign to dislodge the Iraqi forces from Kuwait began in September "though [the government was] stating publicly that the only mission was to defend Saudi Arabia and enforce UN sanctions." It would be interesting to learn if such intuitives had been sensitized to the need to discover truth in childhood within families where lying and denial were the collective norm. One woman with such a history returned from an October vacation in a panic because she had seen solar light refracted as sun dogs in the sky and was convinced that they meant war was imminent. When others dismissed her intuition as "ridiculous," she reexperienced the childhood feelings of shame for seeing what others failed to see. In therapy, she was able to accept her intuition as accurate, enabling her to probe her Cassandra-like powers and the family patterns that had made her so untrusting of outer authority and even her own sight.

2. Yael Haft, personal communication.

3. These extraverted and active levels are reflected in the Celtic mythology of war goddesses, who fought with swords and shields, trained heroes in feats of skill, and challenged them as lovers and adversaries to prove their strength.

4. This belief in the animism of tools is ancient and widespread. Celtic warriors believed their swords could even sing of the battles they had fought.

5. That my own clients tended to have strong reactions to the war and its images may have been influenced by my own involvement in the war. It is possible that the holding environment in the transference/countertransference field in my practice was more permeable than that of some of my colleagues, who had no immediate and personal concerns with individuals and issues on both sides of the conflict in the Gulf area.

6. This part is sometimes experienced as a walled-off layer into which the fragile ego collapses. But in more developed personalities, it is more often felt to be a pocket that has been disidentified from and lived around. When the pocket's chaos is experienced, the rest of the functioning personality can support this to some extent. In many creative individuals, access (via mood shifts induced by emotion, mind-altering substance, meditation, etc.) to this pocket is considered valuable as a source for imaginal work.

7. This word may mean "loss."

8. Transformation in this realm does not connote development as it tends to when we use the term today. Rather it connotes the changes of shape or form that the underlying essence undergoes throughout the life, death, and regenerative cycles. It is closer to shapeshifting and the psychoidal levels of psyche, not to the development of consciousness.

9. These forms include extrasensory perception, participation mystique, out-of-body, and near-death experiences, dreaming and imaginal and subtle body mentation, and awareness of synchronicity. Neumann, already in 1952, pointed to the need to explore such "extrane psychic systems" of awareness (or "field knowledge") that lie beyond ego-consciousness and which we therefore have tended to call "unconscious."

10. This gift is similar to Athena's gift to Asklepios of two phials of Medusa's blood — one to raise the dead and one to destroy. It is similar also to the moon blood of women which brings life or death (Walker 1983, p. 629).

11. Valkyries, too, took the form of ravens to drink the blood of the slain, which was called "the raven's drink" (Walker 1983, p. 847).

Book Reviews

Three Works by Thomas H. Ogden

Jean Kirsch

Projective Identification and Psychotherapeutic Technique
Northvale, N.J.: Jason Aronson Inc., 1982.

The Matrix of the Mind: Object Relations and the Psychoanalytic Dialogue
Northvale, N.J.: Jason Aronson Inc., 1986.

The Primitive Edge of Experience
Northvale, N.J.: Jason Aronson Inc., 1989.

I first encountered the work of Thomas Ogden in his third and most recent book, *The Primitive Edge of Experience*. From its opening paragraph to its final page, his fresh ideas and their clear presentation excited and taught me. He gives shape and coherence to observations of interpersonal dynamics I, too, have made. He articulates a map of the intrapsychic landscape that corresponds to terrain I, too, have explored

Jean Kirsch, M.D., is an analyst in private practice in Palo Alto, California, a member of the C. G. Jung Institute of San Francisco, and a member of the volunteer clinical faculty at the Stanford University School of Medicine.

and could name in general Jungian terms, but which I have not charted in ways that are clinically useful.

I began to wonder how his concepts had developed. Mainly, I was curious about the origin of his idea that there is a sensory floor for all experience which is present from the beginning of psychological development and is active throughout life. Consequently, I looked into his earlier works, *Projective Identification and Psychotherapeutic Techniques* and *The Matrix of the Mind*. As I read I began to think of Ogden as a young man. His style manages to convey not only a depth of experience but also a lively curiosity about the human mind and body, along with a genuine desire to relieve suffering that one often finds in medical students and residents. The way he writes about people shows a very special quality of kindness and intelligence. His kind intelligence illuminates every case presentation, every concept, and is certainly extended to those of his colleagues whose work he integrates or challenges.

Ogden sustains a playful tension in his diction. Words like *interplay, interrelation, interactive*, and *linkage* crop up with regularity through all his articles and books. Language is "a responsively flexible medium [that] create[s] a transitional realm of experience" (1982, p. 106). His books are a re-creational amplification of Winnicott's potential space. Like so many contemporary thinkers, he is caught by Hegel's concept of the dialectic, "a process in which each of two opposing concepts creates, informs, preserves and negates the other, each standing in a dynamic (ever-changing) relationship with the other" (1986, p. 208). Not only is this concept central to the development of his ideas about psychological growth and function, it is central to his way of thinking and writing.

Like Jung, Ogden developed very early in his career an interest in and an unusual capacity to relate to seriously disturbed schizophrenic patients, an interest and capacity he sustained throughout his psychoanalytic training. When classical theory proved inadequate to explain his observations, he turned to the works of Klein, Winnicott, Bion, and Fairbairn. By integrating, modifying, and ultimately expanding their ideas, he created a bridge between psychoanalytic instinct theory and Klein's concept of the infant's phylogenetic inheritance.

To this end, he drew upon Chomsky's theory of linguistic deep structures with its underlying assumption that "human beings do not randomly organize experience," but rely upon "preexisting systems for organizing that which is perceived" (1986, p. 13). As both Solomon

(1991) and Stevens (1982, p. 44) have demonstrated, Chomsky gave to the field of linguistics what Jung had earlier provided psychology with his theory of archetypes.

Ogden stands in relationship to classical psychoanalytic theory as Fordham does to analytical psychology, each in his way engaging in a dialectic with a remote standpoint, i.e., the Kleinian. Neither Fordham nor Ogden views psychological development as a linear process by which the individual arrives at a fixed level of maturity. Rather, both recognize that mature levels of development are in constant interplay with earlier, more primitive levels. Fordham proposes that the Self, the totality of the psyche, has both integrative and deintegrative functions, which are in constant operation. However, Ogden takes a different tack, and it is here that he is truly original. His experiences with extremely regressed patients convinced him that the schizoid condition does not represent our most primitive psychological state, but that it is contiguous with an inarticulate sensory realm where data is organized and behavior is driven in even more archaic schemes. This primitive edge between the schizoid and what lies beyond it is a generative zone, as vital as the borderline between the depressive and the schizoid conditions.

Thus, in addition to the Kleinian notion of the two basic psychological positions, the paranoid-schizoid and the depressive, he theorizes a third, which he calls the autistic-contiguous position. Rather than tying these positions to a developmental timetable and assuming that one supplants the other, he proposes that the three positions coexist at all levels of maturity, and that access to earlier phases of development is the mark of the fully functioning personality.

Consequently, psychopathology consists of what he calls a "collapse" into one position or another, from which the individual attempts to relate to his inner and outer experience in a fixed and rigid way. The autistic-contiguous position is that state of being which serves as the "sensory floor of experience." It is this innovative idea which opens the door to understanding phenomena that are readily observed both in and out of the psychotherapeutic setting. To my thinking, it offers the possibility of a theoretical grounding for such techniques as sand play, dance, movement, and art therapy, techniques which many analysts consider nonanalytic, or extra-analytic at best.

Having briefly summarized Ogden's work and having indicated the position I see him occupying in relationship to analytical psychology. I would like now to review in turn each of his books, with special emphasis on the third, in order to trace the ideas constellated in his concept of the autistic-contiguous position.

In the first few chapters of *Projective Identification and Psychotherapeutic Technique*, Ogden gives us a superb description of projective identification, a clear discussion of clinical technique, and a historical overview of the subject. In the last half of the book, there is a fascinating presentation of his observations and treatment of profoundly disturbed schizophrenic patients. He puts forth in great detail and with convincing clinical substantiation several ideas about the way in which the mind operates to generate meaning and to create symbols. He begins to demonstrate a dialectical mode of thinking in his reappraisal of transference and countertransference in light of his experiences with severely disordered patients:

> I have come to view transference as one facet of a two-person transference-countertransference system. Within that system, neither element can be meaningfully understood in isolation from the other. (1982, p. 82n)

This is in contrast to the classically psychoanalytic view of transference and countertransference as exclusively intrapsychic and unrelated.

Crucial to understanding the interactive nature of transference and countertransference is the phenomenon of projective identification — and Ogden stresses that it is indeed a clinical phenomenon, like transference, occurring ubiquitously both in and out of the therapeutic setting. It is a neutral concept, also like transference, an idea belonging to all schools of thought, which will be handled in treatment according to the theoretical orientation of the individual therapist.

> Projective identification is a concept that addresses the way in which feeling-states corresponding to the unconscious fantasies of one person (the projector) are engendered in and processed by another person (the recipient), that is, the way in which one person makes use of another person to experience and contain an aspect of himself. The projector has the primarily unconscious fantasy of getting rid of an unwanted or endangered part of himself (including internal objects) and of depositing that part in another person in a powerfully controlling way. The projected part of the self is felt to be partially lost and to be inhabiting the other person. In association with this unconscious projective fantasy there is an interpersonal interaction by means of which the recipient is pressured to think, feel, and behave in a manner congruent with the ejected feelings and the self- and object-representations embodied in the projective fantasy. In other words, the recipient is pressured to engage in an identification with a specific, disowned aspect of the projector. (1982, pp. 1–2)

This is the phenomenon that the anthropologist Levy-Bruhl described as *participation mystique*, and which Jung recognized early on as a common feature in psychic function. Ogden makes reference to neither. However, he is clinically astute in the way that he elucidates its occurrence in the therapeutic relationship and demonstrates effective therapeutic techniques for holding this kind of projective activity. Drawing upon the work of Malin and Grotstein (1966), he views projective identification as a three-phase operation. The first phase happens within the projector, for whom a part of the self is experienced as either valuable and in danger of attack by other parts of the self, or is itself experienced as so dangerous and threatening that it seems impossible to contain.

Phase two is interpersonal; the projector engages in an interaction with the chosen recipient of this endangered or endangering part, acting in unconscious or partly conscious ways to exert real pressure on that person to think or act in a specific, intended way.

Phase three is both intrapsychic for the recipient and interpersonal; the operation is successful and the recipient does experience a version of the feelings intended. Because the recipient has a different personality structure, the feelings do not have the same meaning and are not handled in the same way. Through the recipient's different handling, the projector may learn to live more easily with that part of the self.

A patient of mine recently demonstrated most clearly the operation of projective identification in her marriage. Describing an interaction with her husband, she said, "I was frantic over that little thing, and I couldn't rest until I had put all my feelings into J., until he felt just as frantic as I did. I thought if he knew exactly how I felt, then next time he'd listen to me and not treat me that way again. I acted just the way my dad used to act with us kids and I hate it."

Projective identification, as formulated here, is a process that serves as: (1) a type of defense by which one can distance oneself from an unwanted or internally endangered part of the self, while in fantasy keeping that aspect of the self alive in the recipient; (2) a mode of communication by which the projector makes himself understood by exerting pressure on the recipient to experience a set of feelings similar to his own; (3) a type of object-relatedness in which the projector experiences the recipient as separate enough to serve as a receptacle for parts of the self but sufficiently undifferentiated to maintain the illusion of literally sharing the projector's feeling; (4) a pathway for psychological change by which feelings similar to those which the projector is struggling with are processed by the recipient, thus allowing the projector to identify with the recipient's handling of the engendered feelings. (1982, p. 36–37)

The seeds that later grew into his formulation of the autistic-contiguous position lie in his discussion of projective identification as a component of all adult object relations in which "primitive nonverbal modes of relatedness persist as the coenesthetic background for diacritic modes of interpersonal communication." The term *coenesthetic* refers to "visceral modes of perception based on the autonomic nervous system" and the term *diacritic* to "higher-level cognitive processes and conscious thought" (1982, p. 70). Early in the development of his ideas, Ogden recognized the continuous and vital activity of earlier modes and more primitive strata into maturity.

In the last half of *Projective Identification and Psychotherapeutic Technique*, Ogden moves into a discussion of the nature of schizophrenic conflict and puts forth his own notions that the schizophrenic patient is driven by unmanageable internal conflict to attack his own capacity for deriving meaning, attacking to the point at which he achieves a state of what Ogden calls "nonexperience," where:

> there is a progressive reduction of fantasy activity of all types (including the type of projective fantasy central to projective identification) and a virtual absence of the type of interpersonal pressure characteristic of projective identification. (1982, p. 141)

He observed in his inpatient work with severely regressed schizophrenic patients that they reached a stage beyond which communication, even via the primitive mode of projective identification, ceases to occur. Drawing from Grotstein's idea of "connative suppression," which describes "the schizophrenic's attack on his own thought processes," Ogden proposes a model of schizophrenia that "takes as its focus the interplay between the level of psychological meanings and the level of capacities involved in generating these meanings." Here we witness how Hegel's idea of the dialectic process influences his intellectual approach to the problems posed by schizophrenia.

This kind of subtle interplay is developed further in his second book, *Matrix of the Mind*, in which his stated goal is to bring the concepts of Klein, Winnicott, Fairbairn, and Bion into the mainstream of psychoanalytic thought (their absence having led to "a depleting form of self-alienation in psychoanalytic thinking" (1986, p. 4)). Looking at psychoanalytic theory as if it were his analysand, he suggests that, similar to the way a person is depleted when he ignores or devalues experience generated in more primitive modes, so psychoanalysis with its dialogue within a body of knowledge suffers if it makes a scapegoat of and exiles nonorthodox analysts. Therefore, he holds and processes the ejected material of object relations theorists, then re-presents them to his psychoanalytic colleagues in a form that they might accept. The result is a felicitous and pertinent account of this important body of thought.

Considering the magnitude of his challenge, to make object relations theory palatable to classical psychoanalysts, one rightfully can not fault Ogden for slighting analytical psychology when, in the process, he elaborates concepts which are almost transparently those of Jung. Nevertheless, one cannot help wishing that he had been able to take that extra step to acknowledge psychology's debt to Jung's genius.

In fact, Ogden's attributions are diametrical. In line with classical thought, he sees the unconscious as personal, its contents a registry of inner and outer experience. He strives to be psychoanalytically correct when trying to account for the autonomy an internal object can assume. Trying not to fall victim to the charge of what he terms "demonology," he twists and turns through an impressive series of mental gymnastics to demonstrate how the ego splits and identifies with an internalized object representation, hence allowing the logical possibility for two active internal agencies of thought and feeling to engage in relationship.

> In brief, internal objects are subdivisions of the ego that are heavily identified with an object representation while maintaining the capacities of the whole ego for thought, perception, and feeling. Such a proposal goes no further in the direction of demonology than did Freud in describing the formation of the superego. . . . The dynamism of an internal object must in every case reflect the fact that an aspect of the ego has been split off and is at the core of the new structure. The fact that this structure (the internal object) is experienced as nonself is accounted for by means of its profound identification with the object. (1986, p. 150)

To invoke Chomsky's theory of deep structure with its assumption that "human beings do not randomly organize experience" but rely upon "preexisting systems for organizing that which is perceived" (1986, p. 13) at this point would carry him perilously close to Jung's theory of complex and archetype, though this is indeed the most economic way to understand the psychological evidence. In fact, he approximates the theory of Perry (1970), later expanded by Beebe and Sandner (1982), of the bipolar complex when he writes, "I propose . . . that internal object relations be thought of as paired, split-off, and repressed aspects of the ego. These paired aspects of self (the internal object relationship) are viewed not simply as self and object representations, but as paired suborganizations of personality capable of semi-autonomously generating experience" (1986, p. 6).

Despite his neglect of the contributions of analytical psychology, I deeply appreciate his reading and interpretation, especially of the work of Klein and Winnicott. The manner in which he structures the reader's experience of this material is so subtle and organically directed that one only gradually becomes aware that the unfolding intellectual argument recapitulates the very process of psychological development that he is describing.

There are many ways in which one might review the substantial book, *Matrix of the Mind*, but since my aim is to progress toward the concepts he developed subsequently, I will focus now upon that material which grounded him for the next step in his thinking. His earlier observation that in severe phases of schizophrenia his patients reached a state of nonexperience led him to postulate that there is a level of mental pathology which is no longer psychological, a state so profoundly devoid of fantasy, thought, feeling, and relatedness that meaning has been totally "foreclosed."

Synthesizing the ideas of many analysts (while scrupulously and generously citing his sources), he develops a tri-level classification of psychopathology built upon his conceptualizations of the paranoid-schizoid and the depressive states of being. The highest level of psychopathology is one of conflicted personal meaning. The individual will suffer a neurosis when his "desires . . . are experienced as painfully incompatible" (1986, p. 102). Such a person has developed a strong enough sense of subjectivity to experience his desires as his own, has acquired a symbolic attitude, is able to preserve parts of himself intact through defenses like repression, and has the capacity for relationships with whole objects. "In Kleinian terminology, this is the psychopathology developed in the depressive position" (ibid.).

The middle level consists of all other recognized forms of psychopathology, the most paradigmatic being the psychoses, which Ogden views as "problems of balance and intercommunication between depressive and paranoid-schizoid modes." He includes here "borderline conditions, pathological narcissism, severe character disorders, psychotic depression, manic-depressive illness, and perversions" (1986, p. 103). At this level of psychopathology the individual's personality development is roughly equivalent to the paranoid-schizoid position, i.e., experience is not interpreted from a stable sense of subjectivity and the predominant mode of symbolization . . . is one in which the symbol and the symbolized are emotionally indistinguishable since there is no interpreting self to mediate between symbol and symbolized . . . events are what they are, and interpretation and perception are treated as identical processes. (1986, p. 61)

The third and lowest level of psychopathology is the one he observed in his most-regressed schizophrenic patients:

This is the realm of "nonexperience" in which potential thoughts and feelings are neither attributed symbolic meaning as they are in the neuroses, nor given existence as things as they are in the psychoses. Examples of this level of disturbance include psychosomatic illness, alexithymia, and schizophrenic nonexperience. The person exists but, to the extent that he has foreclosed meaning, he is psychologically dead. . . . *It must be kept in mind that all three levels of psychopathology are present in every individual, and therefore that psychosomatic foreclosure of meaning may be a feature to consider in the treatment of both the neurotic and the psychotic patient.* (1986, p. 103–104; italics added)

Ogden's tri-level conceptualization of psychopathology ties a form of illness to the level of personality development attained by the individual, and his formulation seems to cry out for a third position to achieve a symmetry of ideas. Although he cites the work on autism by Bick, Melzer, and Tustin in *The Matrix of the Mind* and recognizes the kind of prepsychological body sense that must exist in the state of being associated with the lowest level of pathology, his ideas have not yet consolidated to the point of formulating the third position, the autistic-contiguous, which is the focus of his third book.

I cannot emphasize enough the importance of the dialectical process both to Ogden's view of psychological development and to the development of his ideas about how the psyche develops. Play, in Winnicott's sense, is crucial to the dialectic.

I have proposed that Winnicott's concept of potential space be understood as a state of mind based upon a series of dialectical relationships between fantasy and reality, me and not-me, symbol and symbolized, etc., each pole of the dialectic creating, informing, and negating the other. The achievement of such a dialectical process occurs by means of a developmental advance from the "invisible oneness" of the mother-infant unit to the subjective threeness of the mother-and-infant (as symbolic objects) and the infant (as interpreting subject). (1986, p. 231–232)

Analytic space is constituted analogously to the potential space that develops between the mother and child. The developing child/analysand depends upon the capacity of the mother/analyst to successfully receive and process his projective identifications in such a way that the dialectic is sustained and the play/analytic space for imaginative construction of meaning is preserved. This is certainly akin to the dynamics Jung discovered were central to the individuation process: a tension of opposites generates psychic energy and, by evoking what Jung calls the transcendent function, gives rise to an unpredicted element, the *tertium non datur* (the third not given), that surprising and creative development one so often encounters in analysis. An analytic attitude which supports endurance of the tension between psychological opposites makes space for the possibility of unexpected connections.

For Jung and analytical psychologists following him who consider the religious function a normal and essential part of psychic life, this opening in the analytic space allows for the entry of the transpersonal dimension. Ogden is again like Jung in his recognition that projective identification is contrary to play because of its powerful demand upon the recipient/analyst to think, feel, and act in a highly specific way. Jung recognized that a state of *participation mystique* between analyst and analysand could preclude growth.

It may be useful to point out here the difference between Jung's usage of the word *dialectic* and Ogden's. They do not refer to the same thing at all. Ogden employs the term with reference to an interplay of ideas, feelings, concepts, stages of personality development, etc. Jung, on the other hand, uses the term to mean both the face-to-face relationship with equal exchange between analyst and analysand (which he thought was the suitable mode of conducting an analysis) and an intrapsychic dialogue between ego and the unconscious which he thought was the essence of psychotherapy.

The Primitive Edge of Experience is Ogden's major work, wherein he makes two significant contributions to psychoanalytic thought. The first is his formulation of the third and most basic level of personality development, the autistic-contiguous position. The second is his elaboration of the dialectic process abiding at the very marrow of psychological growth.

The book itself has an interesting structure. He opens and closes with an almost philosophical discussion of the tension between knowing and not knowing, out of which psychoanalytic thought itself emerges.

> The psychoanalyst is . . . a student of that which cannot be known. It is little wonder that we cling to our ideologies, our patriarchs and matriarchs, our analytic heroes and heretics, and our analytic schools, all of which serve us in our efforts to avoid awareness of our own confusion. (1989, p. 2)

His introductory comments address the anxieties one feels approaching a new text: the reader's state of knowledge is challenged; in some yet-to-be-discovered way, he or she will be altered by the encounter with this book. He closes with a chapter entitled "Misrecognitions and the Fear of Not Knowing." Here he elucidates how "substitute formations are utilized to create the illusion that the individual knows what he feels." While these illusions "help to ward off the feeling of not knowing, they also have the effect of filling the potential space in which feeling states (that are experienced as one's own) might arise" (1989, p. 221). In structuring the reader's experience of his material in this way, he draws a protective and relativistic circle around his own ideas, suggesting that when anxiety arises in confrontation with the text, he or she might tend to ward off new understanding by insistence on old doctrines. Simultaneously, he offers up his ideas for their inevitable reconstruction as they are integrated and translated anew in our thoughts and feelings.

Ogden proposes that we structure our experience in particular ways. Raw sensory data, input from the external world and the unconscious mind, are processed through what he calls "modes," which have specific qualifying functions. He describes three basic modes which continue to operate throughout life: the depressive mode, the paranoid-schizoid mode, and the autistic-contiguous mode.

The psyche malfunctions, i.e., psychopathology manifests, when one of the three modes dominates the way all experience, inner and outer, is structured—in his words there is a "collapse" into one of the three positions, or modes. The psyche functions normally and growth occurs when there is an active dialectic between the three modes, when there is a potential space between the three in which thoughts and feelings can exist in playful and potentially creative interaction. Thus, each of the three modes, in dialectic fashion, "creates, informs, preserves, and negates the other, each standing in a dynamic (everchanging) relationship with the other" (1986, p. 208). Additionally, psychopathology manifests in specific ways when there is a collapse into one mode.

There are four specific qualifying functions of each mode: (1) its form of symbolization; (2) its method of defense; (3) its quality of object relatedness; and (4) its degree of subjectivity.

In the depressive mode, the individual is fully able to utilize and create proper symbols; the symbol re-presents that which is symbolized and stands separate from it. One's method of defense enables one to contain painful experience; through repression and related defenses unacceptable portions of experience are shut away whole and intact. There is historical continuity to object relationships, ambivalence is tolerated, and others are subjects who can be harmed. The individual has a firm sense of "I-ness," with the capacity to interpret perceptions and create meaning. If unopposed, the depressive mode leads to certainty, stagnation, closure, arrogance, and deadness; one becomes isolated from bodily sensations and from lived experience (1989, p. 29–30).

Ogden sees value in the paranoid-schizoid mode since experience structured in this mode will split linkages and open closures, leading to the possibility of new thoughts and feelings (1989, p. 30). If unopposed, however, it leads to fragmentation of thought, discontinuity of experience, splitting of self and object, and to a psychic state in which one is "buffeted by thoughts, feelings, and perceptions as if they were external forces or physical objects occupying or bombarding oneself" (ibid., p. 23).

Psychosis is paradigmatic of this position, but it also gives way to a wide range of pathologies including borderline and narcissistic personality disorders. The individual functioning in the paranoid-schizoid position does not symbolize properly, but makes symbolic equations in which the symbol and symbolized are emotionally equivalent. The chief method of defense is splitting: "one secures safety by separating endangered from the endangering" (1989, p. 22). Projective identification is heavily utilized, both as a defense and as a way of relating to others. Object relationships tend to be brittle and unstable; history is always being revised. Both the self and the other are viewed as objects. Hence, subjectivity is rudimentary; no interpreting subject stands consistently between perceptions and what is thought and felt about those perceptions.

Finally, the autistic-contiguous mode provides the "bounded, sensory floor of experience through rhythmicity and continuity of sensory experience." At this level, experience is processed presymbolically, hence preverbally. Defenses are chiefly in the form of self-soothing activities which, although they are under conscious control, can impose tyrannically since the individual may be absolutely dependent upon them to protect himself from a formless, nameless dread. Relationships to the object are tactile, the relationship of shape to the feeling of enclosure, of beat to the feeling of rhythm of hardness to the feeling of edges (1989, p. 52–59). Countertransference responses to individuals processing experience in this mode are likely to be somatic.

Subjectivity in the autistic-contiguous mode does not exist as a psychological phenomenon *per se*, but rather is a nonreflective state of "going on being." If structuring of experience through the autistic-contiguous mode is unopposed, i.e., balanced in dialectic process by either or both of the other two modes, it can lead to "a machinelike tyranny of autistic defenses which are sensory-based escapes from formless dread." Psychosomatic illness is one pathological manifestation, as well as the schizophrenic state of nonexperience described above. Anxiety experienced in the autistic-contiguous mode "involves the experience of impending disintegration of one's sensory surface . . . resulting in the feeling of leaking, dissolving, disappearing, or falling into shapeless unbounded space." This stands in contrast to the anxiety generated in the depressive postion, which "involves the fear that one has in fact or in fantasy harmed or driven away a person whom one loves" and to paranoid-schizoid anxiety that "is at core a sense of impending annihilation . . . experienced in the form of fragmenting attacks on the self and on one's objects" (1989, p. 67–68).

What can it mean that each of us carries within us the apprehension of our own psychological disintegration, only manifesting in pathological states of mind, yet always present at an unconscious level? The possibility of fearing dissolution must itself be archetypal, hard-wired into the psyche, a deep structure, and as such must have adaptive significance. This archetypal process of disintegration must be the basis of what Freud recognized as the death instinct and what Fordham calls the deintegrative function of the self. Perhaps it is the psychological equivalent of physiological catabolism (breakdown by metabolic process) which, in balance with anabolism (constructive metabolism), is fundamental to life processes. Certainly, it is a central element in all processes of psychological transformation, a fact recognized by the alchemists and incorporated into the universal and archaic practices of shamanism.

In naming this third and most primitive mode of structuring (and now we might add "destructuring") experience, Ogden uses the term *autistic* because of his belief that in pathological autism the same defenses, ways of experiencing meaning, and engaging in object relations are to be seen in hypertrophied form. He uses the term *contiguous* since "the experience of surfaces touching one another is a principal medium through which connections are made and organization achieved in this mode" (1989, p. 50). It is worth mentioning, parenthetically, that the three modes of Ogden are somewhat analogous to Jung's three stages of consciousness: the anarchic or chaotic, the monistic, and the dualistic. The problem Jung presents is similar to Klein's in that he ties his stages to a developmental timetable, the chaotic spanning childhood, the monistic occurring in adolescence and early adulthood, while the dualistic stage is reached in maturity.

Ogden's second major contribution to psychoanalytic thought is his elaboration of the meaning and experience of the dialectic process in the analytic setting. He is particularly careful to observe in detail the intrapsychic and interpersonal steps through which the individual makes the transition from one level of development to the other. His investigations, his reporting of interactions and of feelings and thoughts which are stirred in himself, of fantasies and external events, his own and his analysands, his supervisees and their patients, lead him to formulations that are essentially those that Jung himself made. Compare, contrast if you will, these two passages, the first from Ogden, the second from Jung.

> The concept of a transitional Oedipal relationship is proposed as a way of understanding the psychological-interpersonal processes mediating the entry into the female Oedipus complex. As is the case with other transitional phenomena, this transitional relationship serves the function of allowing the discovery of otherness in a form that is experienced as both *me* and *not-me* at the same time. In the context of the transitional relationship created by mother and daughter at the threshold of the Oedipus complex, the little girl falls in love with her mother who is unconsciously identified with her own (internal object) Oedipal father. The question of whether the little girl is in love with her mother or father (in love with an internal object or an external object) never arises. (1989, p. 6)

> The process of coming to terms with the unconscious is a true labor, a work which involves both action and suffering. It has been named the "transcendent function" because it represents a function based on real and "imaginary," or rational and irrational, data, thus bridging the yawning gulf between conscious and unconscious. It is a natural process, a manifestation of the energy that springs from the tension of opposites, and it consists in a sequence of fantasy-occurrences which appear spontaneously in dreams and visions. The same process can also be observed in the initial stages of certain forms of schizophrenia (Jung 1943, par. 121)

Ogden has discovered the basic similarity in growth processes, whether in the context of infant–mother or analyst–analysand. It is the same process discovered by Jung and called the transcendent function. He brings us to an awareness that the way a baby grows out of infancy and the way a child accomplishes the transition between preoedipal and oedipal stages of development may be similar to the way a psyche makes the transition from the paranoid-schizoid position to the depressive position, or to the way the psyche individuates at any stage of life. These transitions are accomplished through a natural process that we may describe as a dialectic, or as a tension of opposites. The elements in the dialectic or opposition may be unconscious and conscious, fantasy and reality, *me* and *not-me*. It is a process that is humanly mediated, i.e., it occurs in the context of an interpersonal relationship that has both personal/real and archetypal/fantasied aspects.

However, Jung asserts, and in this respect deserves the title of mystic, that the human voice can sustain a dialectic with the archetypal level itself (his conversations with Philamon), hence transforming both ego and the face of the divinity. (This notion is to be found in the Rig-Veda; Jung makes reference to it in *Psychological Types* (1921): the singer's praise unites with the bull of primordial power to create the Brahman, the essence of divinity.)

Ogden's lively curiosity about what happens at the edges has yielded what I feel is one of the most interesting aspects of *The Primitive Edge of Experience*. He has produced a lengthy elaboration, rich with clinical examples, of the child's transition from the preoedipal into the oedipal stage. Through the obfuscating language of object relations theory in the paragraph cited above, one can observe that once again Ogden has drawn conclusions similar to Jung's, to wit, his belief that the mother's animus, her contrasexual archetype whose content is so directly under the influence of her personal father, is a crucial factor in the child's psychological development. Indeed, this is Ogden's belief as well, and it is illuminating to follow his thinking about the dynamics of this influence.

James Gleik, in his book *Chaos*, writes poetically of the philosopher Theodor Schwenk's conception of the dynamics of approaching turbulence.

> The rolling of eddies, the unfurling of ferns, the creasing of mountain ranges, the hollowing of animal organs all followed one path, as he saw it. It had nothing to do with any particular medium, or any particular kind of difference. The inequalities could be slow and fast, warm and cold, dense and tenuous, salt and fresh, viscous and fluid, acid and alkaline. At the boundary, life blossoms. (Gleik 1987, p. 198)

The same dynamics must apply when contrasting theories come in contact with one another. Schools of depth psychology, generated in proximity and separated by rivalrous certainties, are still linked by their inevitable relatedness in the matrix of the human mind. Within this medium, our inequities are the stuff of creative dialogue, once the

intervening barriers and chasms have been breached and bridged—
provided, of course, that we are able to recognize one another as potential partners. Jungians should expect no professional *coniunctio* in the
near future, nor should Ogden's work be celebrated as sign of an
engagement. But might a clandestine affair be in progress? If so, rather
like Psyche, Ogden seems not to know the identity of his beloved.

References

Beebe, J., and Sandner, D. F. 1982. Psychopathology and analysis. In *Jungian Analysis*, M.
    Stein, ed. La Salle, Ill.: Open Court.
Gleik, J. 1987. *Chaos: Making a New Science*. New York: Viking.
Jung, C. G. 1943. The psychology of the unconscious. In *CW* 7:3–121. Princeton, N.J.:
    Princeton University Press, 1953.
———. 1921. *Psychological Types*. *CW*, vol. 6. Princeton, N.J.: Princeton University Press,
    1971.
Malin, A., and Grotstein, J. 1966. Projective identification in the therapeutic process.
    International Journal of Psycho-analysis 47:26–31.
Perry, J. W. 1970. Emotions and object relations. *Journal of Analytical Psychology* 15,
    1:1–12.
Solomon, H. M. 1991. Archetypal psychology and object relations theory. *Journal of
    Analytical Psychology* 36, 3:307–329.
Stevens, A. 1982. *Archetypes: A Natural History of the Self*. New York: Quill.

Listen to the Voice Within: A Jungian Approach to Pastoral Care
Christopher Perry. London: SPCK, Holy Trinity Church, 1991. 229 pages. £7.99

Reviewed by David J. Dalrymple

This book is a fine introduction to the many ways in which the ideas of Jung's
analytical psychology can contribute to and transform pastoral counseling and
psychotherapy. This book offers a way of understanding the many intricacies of
intrapersonal and interpersonal relationships for those working in pastoral settings.
The author is an analytical psychologist who lives and works in London. He writes
as a clinician rather than as a theologian. He draws on psychoanalytic understanding of early development, believing that Jung's emphasis on spirituality and later
life needs a corrective counterbalance.

Ironically, this book is published at a time when the field of psychotherapy is
increasingly colored by the "the tri-disciplines" (psychiatry, clinical psychology, and

David J. Dalrymple, D.Min. in Psychology, N.C.PsyA., is a Unitarian minister, a Jungian analyst, a member of the Chicago Society of Jungian Analysts, and serves on the board of
the National Association for the Advancement of Psychoanalysis. He is a certified member of
the American Association of Pastoral Counselors and has served as a Chaplain and Clinical
Pastoral Education supervisor in both medical and mental hospitals. He practices in Chicago
and Rockford, Illinois.

social work). These fields have professional guilds which lobby to influence the public's understanding of which profession will wear "the mantle of healing." Which guild will be recognized or reimbursed for treating the emotionally troubled? To its credit, the field of psychoanalysis has honored the multidisciplinary nature of healing, recognizing that many professions mediate psychotherapy, and mental health disciplines can incorporate psychoanalytic knowledge into their clinical endeavors.

In this climate, it is easy to forget that the initiative, the prerogative, and the responsibility for "the cure of souls" were once in the religious community and its pastoral healers. It was the pastor who cared for and contained the developing individual with respect to both the personal and the symbolic dimensions of the soul in its pathos. However, our age is a time when collective religiosity and pastoral ministries often lack a basic theoretical and practical understanding of what is involved in healing. Many clergy continue to ignore the insights of depth psychology, naively misusing religious beliefs, dogmatic responses, and credal answers in order to defend against the individual's experience of the psyche.

It is refreshing to read *Listen to the Voice Within*, an honest and comprehensive effort to relate Jungian approaches to pastoral care: "to show those active in pastoral settings such as parishes, schools, and hospitals how Jung's ideas can help them in their everyday work." Difficult theoretical ideas are illustrated by case examples, many of which illustrate the neurotic symptoms so present in the lives of parishes, pastors, and religious counselors. The question this author poses throughout is, "How can we reconcile relation with the soul to the purposeful use of skill?" How can we professionally care for others without losing track of what beckons from within?

Jung had been similarly concerned that the person mediating healing not ignore his or her own psyche:

> The doctor who has no wish for (analysis) . . . will be found wanting, cling as he may to his petty conceit of authority . . . How can the patient learn to abandon his neurotic subterfuges when he sees the doctor playing hide-and-seek with his own personality, as though unable, for fear of being thought inferior, to drop the professional mask of authority, competence, superior knowledge, etc.? (Jung 1928, 287–288)

The author's journey into Jungian psychology began as he felt the need for "an introductory text that would act as a sort of Ariadne's thread to help him find his way through the labyrinth of the human psyche and its manifestation in relationships and in group and organizational settings." He, like many pastors and counselors, was "searching for a framework within which everyday work experiences could be conceptualised and understood — in other words, that what seemed mystifying and meaningless could be transformed into something comprehensible and meaningful" (pp. 4–5).

The author discusses how Jung's ideas can be helpful in everyday clinical pastoral work. He focuses on subjects such as the pastor's vocation, the developing Self, the tendency to resist change, and the nature of emotional defenses. Case material illustrates the disturbing relationship that often develops between pastor and individuals as well as their institutions. The author has a particular sensitivity to therapeutic opportunities around loss and separation. He emphasizes that attention to dreams forms part of "the spiritual quest." Pastors can befriend their dreams by reflecting upon them, playing with their images, and thinking about the rectifying messages conveyed about the life context of the dreamer. Dream work helps us relate to inner space. We can listen to the voice within by befriending our dreams.

It is not uncommon for clergy and other "helping personalities" to seek Jungian analysis when they realize their "needy selves" should not be projected onto clients and when their persona identifications cut them off from the mutuality of other people as well as from "the voice within." Pastoral roles often create isolation, loneliness, and self-denial as the pastors try to love others. Clergy are particularly prone to anxiety, inadequacy, guilt, and self-criticism, since the reality of their personal identities does not live up to their idealized self-images and vocational expectations. They are often prone to workaholism, depression, angry outbursts, and somatic complaints. This book reminds us that serious damage can be inflicted on parishioners and patients if the shadow material from pastoral one-sidedness is not confronted and worked through.

Listen to the Voice Within refers frequently to the writings of Jung and contemporary Jungians, so it may be too elemental for analysts. It is a basic introduction to Jungian psychology and a valuable resource for those working in the field of pastoral care and counseling. Clergy, religious educators, institutional chaplains, pastoral counselors, students in clinical pastoral education, and seminarians will find this book helpful as they seek a coherent and adequate understanding of neurotic symptoms and their healing. *Listen to the Voice Within* is a helpful invitation for clergy who know they are symptomatic but are hesitant about entering analysis.

Christopher Perry's reflections remind us that the pastoral care and counseling movements do not need to yield the "mantle of healing" to the tri-disciplines which the public has come to associate with psychological healing. The pastoral world is fraught with opportunities for deeper therapeutic intercessions with men and women. This work reminds us that the "cure of souls" begins by listening to the voice within our own psyches.

Reference

Jung, C. G. 1928. The therapeutic value of abreaction. In *CW* 16:129–138. Princeton, N.J.: Princeton University Press, 1966.

Dance Therapy and Depth Psychology: The Moving Imagination
Joan Chodorow. London: Routledge, 1991. 172 pages.

Reviewed by Lee Roloff

When thinking about depression, of recalling its summonings, withdrawals, hidings, silences, mortifications, immobilities, dreads, and abysses, we are not "thinking" at all; we are summoning memories of feelings, of states of being that, at the time of "depressing" the psyche and body, have emptied the cognitive abilities "to name," "to abstract." In a depression, the summonings are images, colors, moods, distortions, contractions. Having been depressed, the urge might be to discuss it, to mull it through, to speak of its inarticulateness. Or we might color it, scumble the paper with darkness of color, slashing the darkness created with vermilion. Or we might try to find the metaphoric language of the depression, as the English poet Patrick Morgan attempts in "Nocturne."

> It is one of those nights tonight,
> when, face to darkness with the ungraspable,
> neither to be, nor not to be, brings
> any succour to the mind . . .
> (Roloff 1973, p. 119)

Or there might be some attempt to select and arrange images in a sand tray that mutely attest to the agony of the inner condition. Expressive arts therapy, bibliotherapy (and its creative ally, poetry therapy), and sand tray therapy all attempt to move the immobile, to express the inexpressible, to image the unimaginable. There is another intriguing possibility: move and dance the body in space and time and do so with a witness to view that "dance of being." Mover and witness, dancer and observer—this is the dyadic complement to analysand and analyst, client and therapist, that Joan Chodorow explores in her important and implicative book.

The essence of Chodorow's sustained essay on psychology and the body and the moving ways of both synchronously in expressive movement is contained in a quotation of Jung that appears in the very last lines of her book: ". . . And so individuation can only take place if you first return to the body, to your earth, only then does it become true."[1] The fullest measure of consciousness is not what we think about ourselves, but rather what we continually find out about ourselves. This matter of the continuing unfolding of ourselves to ourselves is not held and contained by *thought* alone, but by the riskier business of "coming to our senses" through the endless play of imaginal dance and movement that dreams and fantasies contain but, more elusively, by the dance and movement of *emotion* that thought alone cannot elucidate. As Jung himself experimented in the sand by the shores of Lake Zurich, it is what is materialized, embodied, and concretized that

Lee Zahner-Roloff, Ph.D., is professor emeritus of Northwestern University, an analyst in private practice in Evanston, Illinois, and training analyst at the C. G. Jung Institute of Chicago.

reveals what is "moving" one, "shaping one," and inevitably, "organizing one" into the startled sense of selfhood. What Chodorow advances, and does so with cogency and urgency, are the archetypal foundations of image *and* feeling.[2] Or, to put it the other way around, all feelings have an imaginal complement, or body state, that is immediately recognizable and communicable throughout all the world's peoples.

The fundamental emotional states are grief, joy, anger, fear, contempt, shame, and startle. That is, these are the chief expressive actions formulated by Charles Darwin, and his formulation includes the presence of sustained and relatively uniform body movements. Building upon Darwin's early observations, later theorists added the element of interest and its component of curiosity and exploration.[3] For Jung, the embodiment of images is "active imagination," and in the discovery of emotional states through emotional recall and embodiment, it is "active imagination" with the body's discovery of itself and the movement of itself in space and time. As Chodorow reminds the reader, "creative imagination is turned to the creation of the cultural forms: art, religion, philosophy and society; *active imagination* [italics mine] is turned to the creation of the personality" (p. 112).

In *Dance Therapy and Depth Psychology*, the reader is brought into a twofold awareness of just how "the creation of a personality" develops through movement. In one instance, the author herself gives an autobiographical account of how dance and her dance and movement teachers mentored her personality and the directions dance and movement have taken in subsequent years through the silence of print to the transformative reaches of dance and movement. She prefers the term *witness* to designate what is carried by the terms *client* and *therapist, analysand* and *analyst*. It is an elegant term, for it restores to the work of the analyst/therapist precisely what is most important: to be witness to the myriad wonders of psychological life. As she observes, "Lack of depth in the witness will limit the experience of the mover" (p. 29).

If there is an imbalance in Chodorow's work, it is to be found in what appears, at first hand, to be an overlong theoretical stating of the "ground" for her work. When she writes of her own therapeutic work, the prose changes, markedly, and the generative excitement is engaging. And yet, it is to her theoretical formulations that I have returned again and again, grateful for the intellectual overviews and the pointings to literature overlooked. While I find the word *pioneering* to be a touch gratuitous, I can only imagine how useful and powerful this book will be for those unfamiliar with the theory, and far more important, for those not only unfamiliar but ignorant of what dance and movement therapy implies for our work dedicated "to the creation of personality."

Notes

1. The quotation originally appeared in Jung, *The Visions Seminars* (1930–1934) from the notes of Mary Foote. Whether or not these are Jung's exact words is not as important as the spirit which they convey of the inseparable nature of psyche/soma. The fuller quotation appears on page 152 of Chodorow.

2. Chodorow's theoretical grounding in the archetype of image is, of course, the epistemological elements of analytical psychology. Of enormous interest to a reader is her clear and engaging examination of the archetypal nature of feeling in the theoretical works of Charles Darwin, Silvan S. Tomkins, and Louis H. Stewart. While a thorough examination of

these theoretical foundations would be most appropriate, it is impossible to do them justice here. The reader is referred to Chodorow, particularly chapters 8–11.

3. In reflecting upon Chodorow's synthesis of these emotional states, I would suggest that Joseph Campbell's term *aesthetic arrest* is a better formulation of what is termed "interest," simply because it accurately describes the human state in "being taken over," of being "arrested," "stopped," and engaged by phenomena in the world. Whatever the purpose of the archetypal listing of emotions is to remind us, if we need reminding, that these are bodily states as well.

Reference

Roloff, Leland H. 1973. *The Perception and Evocation of Literature*. Glenview, Ill.: Scott, Foresman and Company.

Individuation and Narcissism: The Psychology of Self in Jung and Kohut
Mario Jacoby. London: Routledge, 1990. 267 pages.

Reviewed by Jeffrey Burke Satinover

In one of his *Tales of the Hasidim*, Martin Buber recounts the Zen-like story of a callow young disciple who begs his Rebbe, the *Zaddik*, to teach him the secret of humility. The Rebbe sends his eager student on a series of spiritual misadventures, wherein he learns the utter elusiveness of his goal. When the disciple is at last ready, the Rebbe reveals to him the secret: humility, the quality of character closest to the center of any true spiritual life, is beyond the reach of anyone.

A Christian coda to this story would introduce grace; but in this very Jewish story, grace stands in silence as the crucial, nameless parameter of the disciple's repetitive failures to achieve humility by his own efforts. By its silence, he is directed, when he at last has ears to hear, to God.

Sometime in 1975, a young trainee at an American Psychoanalytic Association (APA) institute in Los Angeles came to visit his brother in Switzerland. Through the English-speaking colony in Zürich, he met some of us American trainees at the Jung Institute. APA analysts at the time were barely tolerant of non-APA Freudians, let alone non-Freudians,[1] and except for a very few oddballs (our visitor was not one) they knew of Jung only as an anti-Semitic mystic, popular among the lunatic fringe (in Los Angeles at the time, this was a very large fringe; now, of course, it's the warp of the main fabric). He was much surprised to find, half a world away, a substantial cluster of Jungian analysts and their trainees who were as enthusiastic and contentious about the jesuitically convoluted writings of an heretical Chicago-based psychoanalyst named Heinz Kohut as were his own fellow trainees and instructors.

High in the Alps during picnics and mountain trips right out of *The Sound of*

Jeffrey Burke Satinover, M.D., is a psychiatrist and Jungian analyst. He is executive director of the Sterling Institute for Neuropsychiatry and Behavioral Medicine in Stamford, Connecticut, and president of the C. G. Jung Foundation of New York. He has been the William James Lecturer on Psychology and Religion at Harvard University.

Music, we excitedly debated Kohut's theories among ourselves and with our visitor, both on their merits and by contrast to the works of our respective masters. Of course, he was unable to assess our critiques of Kohut from the perspective of Jung, since all he knew of Jung was what Freud and Freudians had told him; we were likewise unable to assess his critique of Kohut from the perspective of Freud, since all we knew of Freud was what Jung and Jungians had told us.

Nonetheless, we were all enthusiastic about some of Kohut's ideas and could all identify in our patients—and more importantly in ourselves—many of the motifs Kohut had identified and explicated. This meant that, at last, there was some real common ground between the Freudians and the Jungians. Or, at least, so it seemed.

Mario Jacoby, a Zürich analyst with a markedly "clinical" approach was one of the first Jungians to have discovered Kohut. *Individuation and Narcissism: The Psychology of Self in Jung and Kohut* is the mature summary of nearly twenty years of reflection by Jacoby on narcissism and the psychology of creativity.

Although by no means identified with the London Jungians, the style of Jacoby's thought and writing is as serious and densely learned as is theirs, and he is equally at home as they with the various British neo-psychoanalytic schools. The English translation of *Individuation and Narcissism* is fittingly published by Routledge. But the translator, Myron Gubitz, is an American, and the language therefore lacks both the occasional gracefulness of the best of the English Jungian writers as well as the archness—sometimes full-fledged constipation—of the worst.

The stated purpose of *Individuation and Narcissism* is to detail the similarities between Jung's view of the individuation process and Kohut's view of the transformation of crude into mature narcissism via "transmuting internalization." Many of us who trained in Zürich at the time that Kohut was discovered have made large or small attempts in the same direction (myself included). Jacoby's is by far the best in terms of detail, scholarship, and clinical acumen.

In what has become the ritual introduction to any Jungian essay, Jacoby begins with a chapter on the pertinent myth, in this case the tale of Narcissus and its variations. But like the story of Oedipus as used by Freud, the Narcissus "myth," especially the version by Ovid, is the product of a sophisticated and erudite class of literati within a declining culture.[2] To *base* an archetypal theory of self-esteem upon it would be rather akin to some far-future Jungoid mythologist describing the fantasy lives of children in terms of *Into the Woods* by Stephen Sondheim.

Jacoby, however, doesn't push the archetypal analogizing. Rather, he uses the tale and its variants as a useful but optional backdrop to a succinct discussion of the dual "positive" and "negative" dimensions of the psychology of narcissism. He thereby links Jung's theory of archetypes (with its emphasis on "opposites" contained within a single archetypal pattern) to the divalent view of narcissism recently adopted by many (nonclassical) neo-Freudians.

Narcissism was described by Freud as an infantile precursor of relatedness to others, and he saw it as pathological when predominant in the personality much past infancy. Late forms of narcissism were adopted by the personality as a regressive defense against unconscious conflict. Currently, however, "narcissistic libido" is widely understood by neo-Freudians as a developmental line in its own right. It may be immature, giving rise to pathology, or mature, giving rise to a number of positive character traits. Given this latter understanding, "narcissistic libido" (i.e., libido that has regressively turned narcissistic) is indeed better renamed (by Jung) as "introversion."

Early on, Jacoby tackles the problem of relating Kohut's use of the word *self* to Jung's. His discussion is both compelling and well referenced. Both Kohut and Jung use the term in ways that go far beyond its casual, nontechnical use in classical psychoanalysis. For Freud, the self never needed to be defined carefully because the term was never used technically. The self was thought of as a subjective illusion derivative of underlying drives and conflicts (a kind of semiconscious byproduct of the ego in interaction with the id and the superego). But for both Jung and Kohut, self is in some way real and primary; the features of human personality derive from "it," and "it" exists in some sense before there is any personality at all to speak of.

Kohut and Jung differ, however, in the degree of transcendence they accord to this primary self. Kohut, his intellectual roots in the atheistic, cosmopolitan world of psychoanalysis, says "no transcendence"; Jung, the pastor's son and philosopher of Bollingen, says "lots of transcendence." Yet, even in this they are in a more fundamental accord with each other than even Jacoby realizes: they both try to explain the manifestations of the human spirit (for Kohut, these are primarily wit, wisdom, creativity, and empathy) without direct reference to God. Kohut never mentions Him, even when strikingly religious imagery is evident in his patients' dreams;[3] Jung opts for a more ambiguous position. He claims only that there is an innate psychic "image of God" and that this image is indistinguishable from the Self.[4]

Jacoby devotes the next seventy pages or so to a detailed description of the forms taken by narcissistic libido (introversion) as it matures. He begins here to introduce his own case material and the book takes on a life of its own: the author's voice as an experienced therapist is strong and compelling. In the last third of the book, when he discusses forms of narcissistic disturbance (eschewing DSM III-R categories) and their therapeutic treatment, he is at his best. He leaves the impression of a mature, skillful, and introspective clinician who has found in the intersection of Jung's and Kohut's ideas a congenial subset of theoretical terms with which to express the considerable wealth of his own insight. For this reason in particular, *Individuation and Narcissism* should be a part of every Jungian training curriculum.

Jacoby's maturity as a teacher of others is likewise conveyed by his manner of expressing clinical material: detailed, convincing, sympathetic, and unassuming. The material appears to have undergone little tendentious pruning for publication and "sounds" genuine. The author himself comes across as neither the sometime-arrogant pedant which Kohut appears to have been (gurus of any sort are distasteful; Freudian gurus risk synergizing their conceits), nor as a wannabe wizard, the preferred persona of all too many Jungian adepts of various esoterica, not only narcissism. For Jungians, in particular, Jacoby's book should serve as a healthy antidote to the breathless occultism that too often passes nowadays for good therapeutic technique.

Nonetheless, the book has three major weaknesses. They all lie outside its stated ambition to illuminate the similarity between Jung and Kohut, but within its apparent scope. Clearly, Jacoby's unstated intent is to provide a definitive explication of narcissistic phenomena, and not merely to provide a scholarly illustration of how Jung and Kohut are similar. These weaknesses are, first, that in discussing the psychoanalytic objections to Kohut, Jacoby references, cites, and discusses only *neo*-Freudians; second, that the author does not relate the problems of narcissism to the archetype of (and literature on) the *puer aeternus*; and, third, he fails adequately to address the role of religion in (at least) channeling narcissistic impulses.

To be fair, Jacoby himself is aware of two of these three lacunae. In what reads like a postscript (it's titled "Conclusion"), he states, "I was not able to detail all the subtle elements of [Kohut's] confrontation with the classical psychoanalytic drive theory"[5] and "I focused more on similarities than on differences; as a result I did not, for example, deal with Jung's specific contribution to the psychology of religion."

With regard to the first weakness: I mentioned above that we early enthusiasts felt that in Kohut's work there seemed to be some real common ground between the Freudians and the Jungians. On more careful consideration, this common ground turns out to be not between Jung and Freud, but between Jung and only certain neo-Freudians, Freudians who are already, in some sense, Jungian. These are psychoanalysts whose *political* allegiance remained to Freud, to Freud's followers, and to Freud's followers' institutes (as opposed to one of the breakaway schools) but who have departed from the classical Freudians' rigorous adherence to a reductive model of psychic process.

These neo-Freudians, like the true apostates who broke away entirely, have nearly all turned from Freud's dominant explanatory principle—*unconscious conflict*—to some synthetic or a priori explanation of selfhood, wherein the core organizing principle of the psyche remains inaccessible to analysis proper.[6] Freud would, and did, claim that most of those who rebelled against his ideas—whether remaining within the formal psychoanalytic movement or leaving it—turning instead to some variant of a synthetic or a priori model of the psyche, did so in large part because the narcissistic wound inflicted upon their self-regard by his discoveries was too painful for them to accept.

Freud's argument is infuriatingly self-serving, especially in the context of a discussion of narcissism.[7] But alas, to anyone with even a glimpse of the heights of self-deception to which each of us will rise to preserve his own particular vanity, it is convincing enough. The conflict between "analytic" and "synthetic" models of personality structure is too serious for the merely contemptuous dismissal afforded it by too many Jungians, if not by Jung himself, in the name of just-any-old-"spirit." A Freudian mechanistic universe consisting of nothing but a few large biomolecules stochastically coupling and uncoupling in an enormous vacuum, and thereby incidentally generating an illusory self-consciousness, is arguably preferable to a New Age cosmos stuffed with petty egotisms parading themselves around as gods and goddesses.

The early analysts who made the intellectual break from Freud's ideas because of their reductiveness (but many of whose subsequent behavior lends some justice to Freud's assessment of their character and motivations) included Jung, who was not the first but was by far the most successful in establishing a nonanalytic "psychoanalysis," with a superordinate antecedent "self" as the primary organizing principle of the psyche; Adler, who forced teleology into psychoanalysis under the guise of the will-to-power and its transformation into "social interest" (thereby also turning self-knowledge into a tool of politics);[8] Rank, who began by focusing on artistic creativity as a sphere of human endeavor outside the reach of psychoanalysis but eventually also made "will" the center of his theory of man; Stekel, who hypothesized a kind of supraindividual goal-directed consciousness accessible through universal dream symbols; Silberer, who before Jung saw in both alchemy and dreams a symbolic representation of an innate drive toward ennoblement of character (had he not died by his own hand, he rather than Jung might well have become the modern psychologist of Gnosticism); and, of course, the object-relations schools whose theories propose an inherent maturational drive toward synthesis of parts of the self.

Object-relations theorists are the neo-psychoanalysts most extensively referenced by Jacoby. Their theories are probably the least a priori of all the alternative schools, since "internalized self- and object-representations" are really just mature configurations of the classical drives. Nonetheless, Edward Glover, doyen of classical English Freudians, damns the lot of his object-relations colleagues as—it's the most serious curse he can muster—"Jungian."

All the major departures from Freud, including Kohut's work, have had this in common: they accord to the human spirit an existence sometimes superordinate to, sometimes not superordinate to, but always independent of the biological drives and drive-related conflicts to which Freud was convinced all human mental activity can be reduced. To the classical Freudian, the work of Kohut is merely the latest incarnation of the same old anathema. It started with Adler and quickly reached an apotheosis in Jung, against which all later apostasies can be compared. The true psychoanalyst, devoid of illusion, calmly anticipates that it will raise itself "in every generation" against the stoic abstinence of the genuine Freudian vision. The language changes, but the error remains the same, driven as always by the flight from painful truth to comforting illusion.

The pattern of references in *Individuation and Narcissism*, in its completeness and in its incompleteness, speaks directly to this central contention. Jacoby does make passing reference to classical drive theory in discussing objections to Kohut from other psychoanalysts. But he devotes serious attention and cites almost exclusively the neo-Freudians who belong to the various nonclassical subschools of psychoanalysis. Their work is published mostly in journals such as the *International Journal of Psychoanalysis*, the "big tent" of psychoanalytic publishing. The authors often belong, or are closely tied, to one of the British schools. Following them in their enthusiasm for and objections to Kohut is rather like listening to a cocktail party debate between an Upper West Side Trotskyite and a Los Angeles Leninist: what's needed to make the dinner party is a Wall Street investment banker.

In other words, the only substantially damaging critique of Kohut (and of the neo-Freudians, and of Jung) comes not from Kohut's fellow neo-Freudians, but from dyed-in-the-wool classicists. Barely referenced at all by Jacoby (at least from among the English-speaking authors) are those psychoanalysts who publish mostly in the *Journal of the American Psychoanalytic Association*.[9] Even among its neo-Freudian detractors, this journal is still considered the premier scholarly journal of psychoanalysis in the world. In its pages can be found the most trenchant criticism of Kohut's work. It is also in this journal that the original arguments for and against views of narcissism alternative to the classical were first debated, and in which Kohut himself published the key articles that preceded his books.

Jacoby guesses that Kohut's "critics may feel supported in their views if [he, Jacoby, has] succeeded in demonstrating in a somewhat convincing manner [Kohut's] closeness to Jung's position." Unfortunately, the only convincing critics of Kohut, the classical Freudians, are unlikely to consider Jacoby's work at all, since they read books published by Routledge even less frequently than authors published by Routledge read their work. But if they do, they won't just feel supported, they'll consider it the unintended *coup de grace*.

This first weakness of *Individuation and Narcissism* is not that surprising. After all, there are as few Jungians familiar with classical psychoanalysis (a fair assessment requires both a good experience of analysis, and a certain sympathy for its views) as there are classical Freudians familiar with (a serious representation of) Jungian thought. But Jacoby's failure even to mention the *puer aeternus* is surprising. Zürich is the home of von Franz, she is cited by Jacoby on other topics, and the *puer aeternus* as a problem is endemic to Western culture. It has received a great deal of press, both popular and professional.

It's possible that Jacoby does not consider, or does not recognize, that the problem of the *puer aeternus* is in fact related to the problem of narcissism. But he sets the stage for his own arguments by adducing the popularity of such writers as Alice Miller (*Prisoners of Childhood*). As the title directly suggests, she relates the problems of narcissism to those of a "prolonged infantile attitude" (Jung's original 1911–1912 theory of the formation of the "narcissistic neuroses"). While Miller and the many other writers congenial to the "Adult Child of" sects do not always call it by the name *puer*, they are describing the same phenomenon. Many of them recognize this congruence and some have sought to quote Jungian writers who explicitly describe the problems of narcissism in terms of the *puer aeternus*.

The psychological, and mythological, dimensions of the *puer aeternus* also provide a link to Jung's psychology of religion. The link was already implied by Jung's 1911–1912 description of preoedipal psychopathology in terms of a "prolonged infantile attitude" and its relationship on the one hand to the "introversion of libido" and on the other to the mythological motif of death and rebirth. The mythic background of "narcissism" as named is contained in the simple observation that the Narcissus tale is but one variant of the great Ur-myth of the dying and resurrecting vegetation God, half-human, half-divine, the eternally youthful son, lover, and hero of the Mother Goddess, that originated in the ancient Near East.[10] The story was ubiquitous in antiquity and forms one of the two great chambers (Jerusalem as opposed to Athens) of the living but at present only faintly beating heart of Western culture. Our modern rejection of its truth means — using Jung's canny formulation — that we are able now to experience our God only by acting Him out. He has become the pandemic, ecstatic worship of eternal adolescence.

The story of the young hero's death followed by spiritual rebirth is the universal mytheme par excellence.[11] It is the *leitmotif* of Jung's psychological theory, starting with his break from Freud and ending with his own old-age self-reference as the "Age-Old Son of the Mother"; it drives all the alchemical symbolism he explicated, and it is the key theological story of the West's (and, for that matter, the world's) dominant religion, in both its exoteric and esoteric variants.[12]

The fate of the hero striving for immortal glory is always to meet failure and mortality. This hero is, of course, everyman, each in his own way. Some of these ways seem large to us, some small; some unfold before our eyes, some in the most hidden recesses. It is also the fate of the hero to undergo transformation, of one kind or another, much dependent on how he meets his fate. That transformation may be into a mere shade of his former self, or it may be into the immortally glorified body promised to the humble by faith. For the *narcissi*, who so love their youth they will not let it go, have their reward: their fate is to remain eternally young, lying tanned in cardiac care beds, golden chains caressing their bypass scars. And after death claims them, they will be reborn in flower beds every spring as beautiful ephemera, emblems of human vanity and pride.

With regard to the third weakness, the absence in *Individuation and Narcissism* of a discussion of religion, Jacoby says that he intends only a limited comparison of Jung's and Kohut's theories and practices. But both men laid claim to an overarching and largely overlapping vision of the total human condition. Certainly no one who believes he understands how people can become witty, compassionate, creative, and wise (as does Kohut) can be fairly compared with someone who believes he understands how people can know a neuronally based facsimile of God (as does Jung), without introducing the subject of, well, probably everything, but especially religion.

Serious psychoanalytic criticism of Kohut comes from "below," from the classical Freudians. Not surprisingly, their critique of religion parallels their critique of Kohut and of Jung. Their arguments must be taken the most seriously because they are the most damaging. Their perspective is pure. In their understanding of any aspect of human nature, they eschew all quasi-religious compromises wherein a Godlike psychic entity, whether called "Self" or "self," immune to reduction (analysis), gets smuggled into psychoanalysis by sophistry: they reject Him entirely and all His works. They are determined to construct a wholly human vision of humanity.

On the one hand, as detailed above, *Individuation and Narcissism* does not address the classical psychoanalytic hypothesis that narcissism (both mature and immature) derives from intrapsychic conflict, and that personality matures by making conscious the unconscious dimension of these conflicts, progressively eliminating narcissistic residue and thereby increasing the amount of available object-related libido. But, on the other hand, neither does the book address the opposite hypothesis: that only in partnership with God can man successfully subdue his narcissism. Kohut, therefore, can and should be critiqued from "above" as well, from the perspective of serious, traditional religion. Of course, given the similarity between Jung and Kohut, we may find that Jung, too, is vulnerable from this direction.[13]

The religious view of narcissism is at once subtle and complex, and yet, as the young Hasid in Buber's story came at last to learn, painfully simple. *Individuation and Narcissism* can be read as a convoluted tale of modern moral confusion and adventure. It might have been as brief and elliptical as a haiku. Instead, its plethora of references trace the forays of both Jungians and neo-Freudians in a heroic, eighty-year-long intellectual safari to hunt it down at its den: pride—after all, isn't that what "narcissism" is?—and from this very heart of darkness thence to provide us all with an analytic triptych back home to . . . humility.

Alas, since this quarry is beyond unassisted human effort, the task these theoreticians have set themselves is vain. But like the tantalizing mixture of rumors and fragments of maps, some partially true, some utterly forged, that guide and beguile the treasure hunters of children's tales, their journeys are fascinating in their own right, and they discover much of value along the way. At the end of the quest, we would like our adventurers to admit, as did the greatest of the alchemists, Michael Maier, that they have nothing to show for their labors "but a feather," but they don't.[14]

It was inevitable that psychoanalysis would eventually founder on and fragment over the closely related mysteries of human self-regard and the spirit. If you penetrate too deeply and too honestly into the mystery of the human self, you will inevitably stumble into a demonic pride which human pride cannot overcome. Indeed, the attempt itself becomes but another form of it: Beelzebub cannot cast out Beelzebub. If we have nothing but our own works with which to wrestle this demon to the ground, then we are truly doomed, and all the contending camps of psychoanalysis might just as well lay down their arms — or should we say, raise their banners proudly? — in defeat.

In the end, none of the authors whom Jacoby so expertly presents, neither the two main ones nor the many peripheral ones, really have the big answers to which they all lay claim. They do teach us many important things about ourselves and our patients. And in *Individuation and Narcissism* we learn most from Jacoby himself. For as a group, the picture these mental adventurers present is mostly a wistful, unwitting self-portrait of the vanity of our modern worship of the psyche. The "problem of narcissism" is but the awkward modern way of describing, without reference to Him, what human beings are like when they are without reference to Him.

Picture, if you will, a large crowd of pale philosophers, standing on a plain, each looking only at his neighbor and trying to jump higher than him. From a distance, they look like a plate of popcorn popping. Each believes that if only he tries hard enough, he can fly unassisted, and fly first. With outstretched hands, the angels, unseen above them, look on helplessly, shaking their noble heads in sorrowful bemusement.[15] As Eliot put it, "Humility is endless."

Notes

1. This was before the American Psychological Association's lawsuit successfully forced the American Psychoanalytic Association to accept nonmedical trainees.

2. Ovid was using an older and quite loosely variable tale to write a deliberate, then-modern allegory. At the time he wrote, the empire was riddled with a growing class of unproductive young men much like Narcissus: beautiful, charming, seductive, loved by a certain shallow type of woman (and man), but too self-involved to be available. His tale was a cautionary warning about one aspect of the growing decadence of his society, set within the metaphor of death and transformation familiar to his readers from the mystery cults that then flourished. The analogy to our own time should be obvious.

3. Kohut regularly interprets the archetypal imagery that appears in his patients' dreams as representations of grandiosity.

4. Recent investigations into the lesions associated with temporal lobe epilepsy and confirmed by neurosurgical experiments (which, if performed on cats, would give the animal-rights types apoplexy) have led a number of neuroscientists to propose a location in the brain responsible for religious experience. Stimulate this part of his brain and even Bertrand Russell would have suffered mystical states. The scientists feel bound to emphasize that this discovery in no way supports the validity of religious concepts. That may be true as far as it goes, but it begs the question as to why we are born with such a capacity if, unlike the drives for sex, hunger, and aggression (likewise stimulable in the temporal lobes), it has no object. So determined is he to cling to his prejudices that at least one researcher believes that, although such experiences are illusory, human beings need them anyway, so part of the brain evolved to provide them!

Similarly, to assert that there is an innate God-image in the psyche and yet claim to say nothing of God is a *petit principe* accorded far more substance by Jungians than it deserves.

5. Jacoby would have found that an article of mine published in 1983 does this, among other things. But it was published in the journal of the American Psychoanalytic Association and so it is not cited (see my further comments below).

6. I am here using the word *analysis* as it should be used, meaning the conceptual "lysing" of a seeming whole in order to reduce it to the interaction of its constituent elements at a so to speak "lower" level. The awkward phrase "reductive analysis" is redundant. A proper use of the term *analysis* best applies to classical Freudian psychoanalysis, since from that point of view the impression we have of the self—our own especially—as a goal-oriented and will-directed "entity" is a mere appearance, a useful but illusory construction; the self's seeming wholeness can be "reduced" to the (largely unconscious) interactions (conflicts) of biological drives with each other, with the demands of society, and with the constraints of physical reality. (The biological drives themselves can further be reduced, some would argue, to the self-organizing behavior of complex biomolecules.) In an analogous way, it is but a mere convenience that we think of the air in an expanding balloon as "having" certain "behaviors," as though this "air" were a discrete entity; the "behavior of air" in a closed container is merely the consequence of the behavior of its constituent molecules. Boyle's laws reduce the macroscopic behavior of an expanding balloon to the microscopic behavior of individual molecules in the same way that Freudian analysis explains motivation and predicts behavior (analyzes "the self") in terms of (conflict among) smaller psychic units: the ego, id, and superego.

7. In fact, Freud hinted at just this explanation for Jung's defection in *On Narcissism*. As Jacoby suspects (he is more correct than he appears to know), this 1914 essay was Freud's first formal foray into the territory of narcissistic pathology. It was indeed intended as an explicit psychoanalytic rejoinder to the noncanonical ideas about "introversion of libido" (a.k.a. "narcissistic libido") proposed by Jung in his 1911 and 1912 *Jahrbuch fur Psychoanalytische Forschungen* articles. On the intellectual side, these ideas so thoroughly confirmed Jung's apostasy that Jung hesitated to publish them for many months, finally doing so only at the urging of his wife. In the same year (1914) Freud also wrote his *History of the Psychoanalytic Movement* wherein he explicitly related Jung's defection from psychoanalysis to Jung's narcissistic character pathology.

8. From the beginning, Adler's followers were predominantly social workers. Most of the earliest exponents of this profession found, and many still find, a congenial ally in socialism, and a cryptoreligious expression of their teleos in Marxist eschatology. As late as 1992, little has changed in this: at a recent New York conference on the child, with speakers representative of various analytic schools, the Adlerian introduced her paper on Freud's case of Little Hans by urging everyone to eschew the evils of nationalism now that the (internationalist/socialist) regimes of Eastern Europe have fallen. She didn't quite have the chutzpah to add, "alas."

9. Only one article from this journal is referenced, by Sidney Pulver. The article is seminal but is only one of many equally important ones that preceded and built up to Kohut's theses.

10. Hillman in particular has sown much confusion by his enthusiastically adopted thesis that the *puer aeternus* and the hero are different archetypes, the former primarily "related to" the father, and only the latter to the mother. This convenient conceit greatly helps the person a bit identified with the *puer* to avoid a cold, hard look at his all-too-obvious mother complex. Ask his long line of ex's what they think of the matter.

In a recent memorial to Joseph Campbell (*Quadrant* 14, 2, 1991), Joseph Henderson has further muddied the waters by asserting that the "adept" is yet another archetype different from the hero. It seems to me that recent Jungians flee from the hero because of his tragic fate (as though denying that fate, rather than heightening its tragedy, will help one avoid it—remember Oedipus?).

But I'm also afraid we need a Jungian Occam's Razor: "Archetypes shall not be multiplied beyond the necessary." Or perhaps, a more explicit psychic zoning restriction would do: "No new archetypes after 1951; all subsequent ones must be subdivisions of an existing archetype. Exceptions will be made on a case-by-case basis for diploma dissertations as long as they remain unpublished."

11. Freud's view of the Oedipus complex thus contains a partial truth: he was correct in asserting the theme's universality, but he ignored the last half of the mythic cycle, with its spiritual dimension, and related it only to the biological drives of sexuality and aggression.

12. Rank's short essay, "The Myth of Birth of the Hero," illustrates the commonality behind its most well known variants from different cultures. Christianity's success in so many different parts of the world may be partially attributable to the fact that the story it tells is one which so many other cultures already know in part. Likewise the considerable differences between alchemy and the Church notwithstanding, Western alchemy is essentially esoteric Christianity.

13. Corollary questions are, therefore, also "To what extent does Kohut's work succeed in replacing religion? To what extent does Jung's?"

14. That is, a quill pen, a nicely self-effacing allusion to Maier's prodigious and highly abstruse literary output (particularly pertinent to Kohut's style), and maybe also to Maier's retrospective self-assessment of that output's ultimate weight.

15. As the author of a number of articles on the subject, one of which is alluded to by Jacoby, I must ruefully include myself among this crowd, determined to jump highest, even now, I suppose.

Female Perversions: The Temptations of Emma Bovary
Louise J. Kaplan. New York: Doubleday, 1991. 580 pages. $24.95

Reviewed by Nancy Pilzner-Dougherty

". . . only those works which satisfy both our temperaments and our minds arouse our unqualified admiration. The failure to make this fundamental distinction is a great cause of injustice."

Preface to *dernières chansons* by Louis Boihat

In *Female Perversions*, Louise Kaplan both fails and succeeds to stir the temperament and to satisfy the mind. She promises to reveal the secrets of Emma Bovary's temptations, she flirts with the experience of sensuality and beauty in her use of literary references and poetic language, but in the end she leaves me dissatisfied. While she delivers some important and creative ideas, she fails to gather them into a clear form. The book's most valuable elements are threefold: a definition of female perversion based on female experience and sexuality; a conceptual framework within which to understand that female and male perversions alike are compulsions performed to ensure intrapsychic cohesion, while they differ in fantasy content and symptomatic enactment; and, finally, a cultural perspective to see that perversions mirror social gender stereotypes.

An ambitious and original work, *Female Perversions* is both enlivened and burdened by its scope. In 580 pages of text, one-third are devoted to female

Nancy Pilzner-Dougherty, A.C.S.W., is a senior candidate at the C. G. Jung Institute of Chicago. She conducts a private practice in Birmingham, Michigan.

perversion, one-third to male perversion, and one-third to a ponderous analysis of the major characters in Gustav Flaubert's *Madame Bovary*. Louise Kaplan is a psychoanalyst and author of several books, most notably *Oneness and Separateness: From Infant to Individual* (1978) and is coeditor of the journal *American Imago*. Her perspective was developed and informed in her work with Margaret Mahler.

In style, this work has none of Emma Bovary's sensibility. It tries, but in all the wrong ways. The idiosyncratic prose is sometimes paradoxical, sometimes elegant and even lyrical, but just as frequently it is overworked, opaque, and unclear. Her style clouds rather than illuminates meaning.

Despite the difficulties of the prose, the developmental/object relations perspective is of value. Kaplan's thinking about too-rigid gender stereotypes is also useful in thinking about the perverse complex's cultural layer. Speculation about the archetypal core of the complex, however, is territory uncharted in this text.[1]

Female Perversions provides one of the first full-scale attempts to understand certain female symptomatologies as perverse strategy. Classical psychiatric definitions of perversion refer to a population that is 99 percent male. This classification is the result of identifying the behavioral symptoms as fetishism, transvestism, exhibitionism, pedophilia and incest, voyeurism, zoophilia, and necrophilia. Perversion is defined as an intrapsychic defense mechanism common to both men and women, the difference between the sexes being one of fantasy content. Kaplan argues that culturally defined gender ideals, which are too rigid and narrow, account for this difference.

The author distinguishes perversion from other fantasy contents by its quality of "desperation or fixity" and defines it as "a precondition for arousal." In addition, a perversion is "performed by a person who has no other choices, a person who would otherwise be overwhelmed by anxiety, depression, or psychosis" (Kaplan 1991, p. 10). What differentiates perversion from kinky, experimental, or simply adventuresome sex is the combination of its static conscious contents and the presence of intense unconscious affective pressure.

A perverse fantasy or enactment serves to reestablish psychic equilibrium in a self structure besieged by anxiety and guilt and weakened by preoedipal trauma. Thus, perversion reinstates psychic homeostasis by developing a scenario that symbolically recreates the child's experience of shame, humiliation, and psychic castration. Concurrently, the adult can now identify with the powerful parent, while the fantasy enactment contains the child's experience of vulnerability and rage. Identified with the adult, the person feels a sense of power about the erotic deed. This illusion occludes the potentially debilitating, more primitive affects of terror and shame.

Order is reestablished by the perverse fantasy as it binds unconscious anxiety and rage within the eroticized ritual reenactment. This unconscious affect can be directed toward an inanimate object, toward others, or toward the self. Concurrently and intrapsychically, eros is used to mediate thanatos, "so that an entire history of desire and punishment can be kept secret and unconscious" (Kaplan 1991, p. 34). Since eros is used by the psyche to stabilize a weak self structure, it is no longer available for intimacy.

From my perspective, one way to read through the list of male and female perversions is to notice *where* the bad object is located. What is threatening must be controlled or kept at a distance. Men in this culture have learned to externalize what they fear, while women are more apt to identify with it. The erect penis is the central actor in the male perversion, the bad object is projected onto the fetish or the body of the other.

In female perversions, as in women's sexuality itself, the object is both more diffuse and internal. Most frequently, it is her own body which must be controlled, wounded, dressed as a sexual object ("homovestism"), gorged, or made to vomit. Manifest in women's perversions are the passion, eroticism, and connection to the object inherent in suffering. This keeps a woman aligned with the stereotypical cultural expectation that her desirousness emanates from passive vulnerability rather than proactive desire. It is sexual innocence rather than sexual prowess that female perversions express.

The fixed and desperate compulsive dieting of the anorexic woman recreates for her a childlike body, wards off anxiety, and produces an eroticized high, thus meeting all the criteria of a perversion. Striving for the image of sexual innocence is the *sine qua non* of the anorexic woman. In fact, "good girls who don't want to hurt or bother their parents" is an apt description of many women who adopt perverse strategies. Seen in this light, we can both more clearly understand and empathically relate to a woman who compulsively pulls her hair out (trichotillomania), makes razor cuts in her arms (delicate self-cutting), or stays in a relationship with a battering partner. She is unconsciously managing the split-off pain of her childhood trauma and the concomitant rage. Paradoxically, by directing this primitive affect toward herself, the affect is contained, fortifying her submissive ego ideal of a good, if wounded, girl. This conforms to cultural gender norms and confirms her female identity.

There are a few gems in this long book. It offers a way to detect a perverse strategy by looking at intrapsychic structure rather than myopically focusing on symptomatic enactment. It asks us to consider the destructive impact of narrow gender stereotypes on human development. While Kaplan moves beyond a solely symptomatic focus and considers the perversion's intrapsychic function, she ironically fails to consider how the fantasy may symbolically be expressing the problem of a girl/mother merger. She discusses at length how a problematic boy/mother merger is expressed and managed via a perversion. For a girl child, gender identity relies on identification with a mother. It makes metaphoric sense that an incomplete merger resolution, where the bad object remains diffusely located within the girl's body, would be symbolically expressed by wounding her own body and trying to separate, to rid her body of the mother/other.

Viewed from a Jungian perspective, rigid gender role expectations are a result of intrapsychic splitting and projection at a cultural level. The reality of this phenomenon is reflected in perversion. However, other factors need to be considered: biological differences, family dynamics, and archetypal energies. What might be the archetypal core of a perverse complex? While female perversion symbolically expresses an eroticized and violent unconscious immersion in grief, more frequently, male perversion represents a denial of grief, an identification with the aggressor, and an eroticized violence directed outwards. These are both archetypal patterns.

An ancient Lakota mourning ritual that involves grief and self-mutilation is performed by the newly widowed Stands-with-Fist, in the recent movie *Dances with Wolves*. Ares, Greek god of war, was himself a victim of child abuse and scorned by the gods for his brutality. Yet he was also the consort of Aphrodite. These two archetypal images represent the current gender pattern, but archetypally the opposites do exist. Consider, for example, the archetypal pattern expressed by the Penetentes of Mexico. These are men who reenact Christ's passion in a ritual of grief and self-mutilation. In terms of the feminine, when Lilith was evicted from Paradise, she, too, handled her loss with envy and vengeance. In other words, biology is not destiny in terms of gender. Archetypally, it is not only "feminine" to suffer and grieve and "masculine" to project vulnerability and attack it with rage. While one set of gender ideals may be preferred by culture, archetypal reality provides other options.

There is a contribution here to women's psychology, yet sadly, it is one embedded in the gender stereotype the author decries. The title *Female Perversions* reflects her intent, but Kaplan is paradoxically unable to speak about women without focusing on men. Her analyses of the four male characters in Emma's life, for example, and her commentary on Gustav Flaubert are more extensive and alive than her appreciation of the character Emma. If only the plight of Emma Bovary had really been the dominant theme of this book. How could Emma express desire in a society that wills passivity for its women? Where might her expression of desire have led Emma? Where might women's expression of desire lead culture?

Note

1. There is not a systematic exploration of perversions done in Jungian literature. Relevant Jungian publications are included in the references by the following authors: Fordham, Gordon, Kraemer, Proner, Storr, Wisdom, and Wyly.

A good recent article that considers a Jungian approach to working with perversion is written by Jungian analyst James Wyly. In "The Perversions in Analysis," Wyly explores the following: the acceptance of the perversion in its primitive form, the concretization in the perversion of unresolved early events and the subsequent split-off affect, the required move from concrete to symbolic in the transitional space of analysis, and finally the prospective intent of the symptom in the person's psyche (Wyly 1989).

References

Kaplan, L. J. 1991. *Female Perversions: The Temptations of Emma Bovary*. New York: Doubleday.
Wyly, J. 1989. The perversions in analysis. *Journal of Analytical Psychology* 34:319–337.

The Place of Creation
Erich Neumann. Princeton, N.J.: Princeton University Press, 1989. 398 pages.

Reviewed by John A. Desteian

Between 1952 and 1960, Erich Neumann gave a series of lectures on creativity which have become the basis for this book. Neumann was, himself, an intensely creative investigator of the human experience, extending his focus of enquiry to archaeology, anthropology, ethnology, biology, physics, art, medicine, and other

---

John A. Desteian, J.D., is an analyst in private practice in St. Paul, Minn. He is the author of *Coming Together—Coming Apart: The Union of Opposites in Love Relationships*.

fields too numerous to list. Each enquiry added to his understanding of the human experience, from his uniquely personal perspective, which is at once scientific and rational and mystical and visionary. *The Place of Creation* is a series of six lectures delivered at the Eranos Conferences.

An aging Jung was working on his most important work, *Mysterium Coniunctionis*, at the time Neumann delivered the first of these lectures. The timing is important, because the theme of Neumann's later work on creativity is unitary reality, a formulation Jung also comes to identify in his final work as the *unus mundus*, in *Mysterium Coniunctionis*. Jung wrote:

> If Dorn, then, saw the consummation of the *mysterium coniunctionis* in the union of the alchemically produced *caelum* with the *unus mundus*, he expressly meant not a fusion of the individual with his environment, or even an adaptation to it, but a *unio mystica* with the potential world . . . undoubtedly the idea of the *unus mundus* is founded on the assumption that the multiplicity of the empirical world rests on an underlying unity, and that not two or more fundamentally different worlds exist side by side or are mingled with one another. Rather, everything divided and different belongs to one and the same world. . . . (1955–1956, pp. 537–538)

In *Mysterium*, Jung illuminated a psychic world which transcended opposites, inner and outer worlds as distinct realms. When Jung stopped writing, because of advanced age, it was Neumann who took up the task of investigating and writing about the world beyond the opposites. In the present time, with analytical psychology going in many directions, and theories of dependency and codependency, object relations, neo-Freudian and other psychologies moving in the direction of furthering causal determinism, this newly published book by Neumann is a lonely voice, calling us to see ourselves and the world from a wholly different perspective. Neumann even alludes to the problem of promoting a theory of unitary reality in a world which overvalues sensible proofs:

> It is a question of determining the unity of a reality which can be no longer (or rather, which can be no longer exclusively) divided into an outer physical-biological world and an inner psychic world by means of the polarization of our consciousness. The work of C. G. Jung gave me courage. . . . But let me add that I am responsible for everything I am going to say: at this point one must risk one's own skin. I am unable to adhere to scientific modesty, supposedly a great virtue in our day, and to remain within the confines of what has been proven. (p. 4)

Bearing this context in mind, we can look at the success Neumann has in elucidating his radical theory of psyche and psychic functioning.

Each of the six chapters is an independent thesis, the lectures delivered at the Eranos Tagungen. In the first chapter, Neumann uses Jung's theory of synchronicity to propose a psychological explanation for parapsychological phenomena and, with this proposition, begins to explicate the unitary reality which transcends the inner and outer world dichotomy we have come to take for a given. Drawing on anthropological and ethnological data, he describes what he calls "field knowledge," which is composed of ego-consciousness and "extraneous" knowledge. His examples help to illuminate the issue. In primitive humans, a bird communicates with the man, giving him information he otherwise lacks. Neumann says:

> The knowledge was not present "in" the primitive—for he didn't find it within himself—nor was it, in the sense of consciousness, "outside," for it was not an objective part of the bird, which for us is part of the outer world. Rather, the knowledge emerges as part of the reality-field in which something happened between the primitive and the bird, as if this knowledge itself, like the primitive and the bird, were a part of the field. (p. 16)

Then, discussing to where knowledge can be traced in the biology of the human, Neumann says:

> It follows that we must learn no longer to regard as self-evident that all knowledge is "inner," that is, in our consciousness, in our psyche, in us as a living creature. This becomes especially clear when we remember that inner and outer are categories of our own conscious system and are competent only for its own reality. . . . (p. 16)

The theory of "extraneous" and "field" knowledge is crucial to the development of Neumann's ultimate argument:

> The course of evolution runs from the experience of the outer to the experience of the objective inner world and to "inner being," from the biopsychic via the sociopsychic realm to individuation, from the "great individual" who, as an exceptional personality anticipates development and points out the way, to the "meantness" of every single person. (p. 381)

The above quote is nigh on impossible to understand as a freestanding thesis, but, of course, Neumann has taken an entire chapter each to define, with eloquent prose, impeccable logic, and precise data, the meaning of this assertion. In Chapter Two, "The Experience of the Unitary Reality," Neumann uses the creativity of the artist as an example of the effects of living within a unitary reality:

> In the unity, the totality, which is the distinguishing mark of every work of art, something comes to rest and finds fulfillment which . . . transcends both the purely psychic and the purely mundane dimensions of reality. This is true of all the arts, since they are the symbolic and in all of them a reunion takes place of those elements our ego is constrained to separate. (p. 109)

Then, in Chapter Three, "The Great Experience," he describes not only the numinosity of the energy comprising the great experience, but also the luminosity of the content or product which attends the experience. Then, building on the theme of unitary reality, Neumann says:

> The openness of the creative personality finds expression in a heightened sensibility and in a capacity and willingness to be deeply moved and impressed. The creative personality is equally open to the psyche and to the world and is not so attuned as normal man to the exclusiveness of a partial world, whether this takes the form of a so-called inner, or a so-called outer world. (p. 139)

The great experience which he is describing later becomes embodied in the great individual to which the quote above refers. Along the way, in this third chapter, Neumann also proposes to differentiate matriarchal and patriarchal creativity, pre-ego and post-ego *participation mystique*, and to place the creative principle in humankind within the fabric of "the creative love of the Godhead" (p. 202).

In Chapter Four, "Man and Meaning," Neumann discusses the elements necessary for humankind to find meaning in their existence. In doing so, he explodes the notion that a differentiation can be made between "authentic" and "inauthentic" experience, redeeming, as he does so, the ego function. He places the ego function squarely in the realm of the instinct for self-preservation and, in the process, also gives respect to the defenses which are so important to the preservation of the Self. Meaning, to Neumann, arises out of the ego encounter with the world and the Self, by which the solitary ego, which is like Ialdabaoth in the Valentinian Gnostic myths, becomes an ego-self. In describing the experience of the unity of the ego-self integrity, he says:

> I am saved neither from my ego-ness nor my evil-ness, not even through my own efforts or the experience of my ego-self integrity. But I experience as meaningful the necessity of my ego-selfness, in the form of ego-ness and self-ness in guilt and innocence, and in the finality implied in every moment of my life by my ego-ness and my mortality, this meaning confers a new sort of innocence, which applies to us as well as to the world which is linked with us and was created at the same time we were. (p. 259)

In Chapter Five, "Peace as the Symbol of Life," Neumann enlarges the concept of peace beyond the mere absence of war, conflict, and turmoil because he recognizes too clearly the inevitability of these conditions as expressions of the unitary reality. Instead, he exchanges the word *peace* for "creative dynamic equilibrium," which, he says,

> is a situation in which the equilibrium between inflow and outflow is not only perpetually reproduced and preserved, but which also enables the entity which exists in the state of equilibrium . . . to grow and develop internally and externally on the foundation of this equilibrium, and to expand its living area by admitting into it new territories in which it can live in new ways. (p. 271)

The very definition of peace, in this context, moves Neumann closer to the transition from a search for meaning "out there" in the world, to a "meantness," which is a unity of the individual with his or her world. One of the few criticisms of the book arises out of the discussion of this theme, namely that he continues, as he did in *The Origins and History of Consciousness*, to see development as linear and from a masculine perspective, i.e., proceeding from encounter with the shadow, to encounter with the anima, etc. My own clinical experience has not been nearly so neat as the schema he proposes. On the other hand, the linear process he describes in no way affects the validity of his perception of peace, meaning, and meantness. With the transition from finding meaning in one's existence in the world, to a unity of meantness of world and individual, the "inner being" arises as a state beyond inner and outer worlds.

Finally, in Chapter Six, "The Psyche as the Place of Creation," Neumann combines a masterful study of anthropological, biological, archaeological, and ethnological material to bring into psychological focus the development of psyche from its earliest historical, evolutionary state to the present. It is in this context that he defines the biopsychic realm as the psyche in its strictly biological functioning, at a time in the historical past, before the development of ego and consciousness. He goes on to describe the sociopsychic realm as that later development of psyche during which humankind formed into groups, advanced culture, and became members of a society. By doing so, Neumann places creativity, inner being, and individuation within the context of a unitary reality which is an a priori state of form and formlessness, but also of a destiny which we are compelled to live out. Thus, he can say:

> Anyone who has seen the sequence of self-portraits of Rembrandt will know that in the searching consciousness of his artistic creation Rembrandt was interested not in his "ego," his "I," but in the destiny that was being enacted in the human being who was himself. His real concern was to apprehend the power that was invisibly transforming him, the formless agency that in every phase of his life was changing and remodelling the character of his face. He was interested in making transparent the creative and formative quality that was the living, really effective background behind the foreground of the "objective" human reality and of the "objective" world. (p. 379)

This book, which moves psychology beyond the simple notion that there is an objective outer world, and an objective inner world which is then projected, is not for everyone. An essential part of analytic training, it will be difficult for those who do not have a deep understanding of Jung. I cannot help but wonder at the direction of analytical psychology had Neumann lived beyond his fifty-five years and, during his older years, had pursued even further the mysteries of the unitary reality.

Reference

Jung, C. G. 1955–1956. *Mysterium Coniunctionis. CW*, vol. 14. Princeton, N.J.: Princeton University Press, 1963.